GW00320425

Pregnancy
for Beginners

Roni Jay

Pregnancy
for Beginners

A guide to having the pregnancy you want

white
LADDER

This edition first published in Great Britain 2009 by
Crimson Publishing, a division of Crimson Business Ltd
Westminster House
Kew Road
Richmond
Surrey
TW9 2ND

A catalogue record for this book is available from the British
Library.

ISBN 978 1 90541 0453

Typeset by Julie Martin Ltd
Printed and bound by Legoprint SpA, Trento

Acknowledgements

Many thanks to midwife Sara Warren who kindly read through the manuscript, added useful points, and answered obscure questions. Thanks also to Rachael Stock Anderson who helped develop the original idea for the book, whilst pregnant for the first time with twins. For the insight this gave her, I should also thank Seren and Jasper. Thanks also to Eleanor Turner for her help with the second edition.

Finally I would like to thank Rich, who was more help and support through all my pregnancies than any book – even this one – could ever be.

Contents

Introduction

You realise when you're expecting a baby that – as everyone keeps reminding you – this is probably the most important thing you'll ever do. Well, yes, so it's doubly worrying that you keep being expected to make decisions you feel ill equipped to make. You know that many of the decisions are vital, and yet you've no idea what's for the best. Other decisions may be less essential in the grand scheme of things (when to decorate the nursery, for example, is not actually a life and death matter) but they're still important to you. This is a very emotional time and lots of things that maybe shouldn't be that important will seem so to you. And that's a good enough reason to give them proper thought so that you feel happy and comfortable.

I realise that not every woman goes through pregnancy with a partner. For the majority who do, this book is intended for both of you. The decisions you'll be making will affect both of you and your child, so it's only right you should both be involved. If you don't have a partner, you may find it useful to show the book to the friends or family whose advice you'll be asking to help you take these big decisions.

I've selected the biggest decisions you're likely to face during your pregnancy and set out all the information I can to help you choose the right course for you. There isn't a definitive right or wrong answer and I haven't attempted to steer you in any way. If there were a clear right or wrong there would, by definition, be no real decision to make. So all the options set out here are potentially right. You're just choosing the best one for you. It's your pregnancy, your baby, and only you can know what will work best for your family. All I have done is:

- set out relevant facts
- clarify the options
- explain the pros and cons of each option
- add any other useful things to think about
- give you the deadline by when the decision has to be made
- run through the worst case scenario (a useful decision-making tool)
- suggest questions to ask yourself to help you decide

I'd also like to add that where I have set out pros and cons, the number of pros – or cons – are no indication of the best decision. One strong argument in favour, or against, could outweigh dozens of arguments on the other side. Just as there are all sorts of arguments in favour of jumping out of an aeroplane without a parachute (the view is great, it's exhilarating, it's a mental challenge, you feel much freer than when encumbered by a parachute, you don't have to worry about fitting your harness properly), and only one real argument against.

The important thing over the next few months is that you enjoy the pregnancy as much as you can, and fret about it as little as possible. You want to feel excited, not worried. Decision making can be fun and interesting, but only when you feel equipped to do a good job of it. You need facts, you need information, and you need clarity of thought. I hope this book will give you all of those, and will help to make your pregnancy and birth the most thrilling few months of your life so far.

part one

Decisions about you

1

When to tell family and friends

It's ever so exciting finding out you're pregnant, and it's obviously something you're going to have to tell everyone eventually. Hopefully you anticipate lots of delight and congratulations all round, but sometimes there are reasons why telling people isn't so easy. Either way, you'll need to decide when to break the news.

The options

The risk of miscarriage is significantly higher in the first three months (12 weeks) and many people are wary of breaking the news before they reach this milestone in case they lose the baby and have to tell everyone they are no longer pregnant. So the choices broadly are:

- tell everyone straight away

- tell them once you reach 12 weeks

- tell some now and some after the 12 week milestone

Obviously you could decide to tell everyone when you get to 15 weeks, or to announce it to one friend a day working through your address book in alphabetical order, or other equally personal decisions. However I'm not going there. I'm just sticking with the standard choice – to break the news now, or at 12 weeks.

TELL THEM STRAIGHT AWAY

This is very tempting, and many people go for this option. About one in five pregnancies is thought to end in miscarriage, but many of these happen before the mother even knows she's pregnant. So the odds are in your favour that the pregnancy will last, but the miscarriage risk is still worth taking into account.

Pros	Cons
You can't wait.	If you miscarry you'll have to tell everyone that you've lost the pregnancy.

You can ask your friends' and family's advice when planning if they know about it.	It can make the pregnancy seem more established in your mind if it's public knowledge, which can make a miscarriage harder to cope with.
Although miscarriage is more likely before 13 weeks, problems can happen anytime. So you may take the attitude that there's just no point fretting.	

TELL THEM AT 12 WEEKS

This is the sensible approach (but who wants to be sensible all the time?). It's an insurance policy against the upset of having to deal with a miscarriage publicly. Eighty per cent of miscarriages occur before 12 weeks.

Pros	Cons
If you miscarry, at least no one will know unless you choose to tell them.	You'll have to resist the temptation to tell anyone for several weeks.
You may enjoy having a secret for the first few weeks.	If people don't know, you can't ask their advice on which room to turn into a nursery, which tests to have, or when to tell your boss (see chapter 2). Or garner their sympathy if you're feeling tired or sick.

	It may be that in your case the pregnancy shows early, or the sickness is very obvious, and it may be hard to keep it secret for that long.

TELL SOME NOW AND SOME AT 12 WEEKS

Another option is to tell those closest to you now, but not to make the news more public until later.

Pros	Cons
You can limit the information to those people you'd tell anyway if you miscarried.	You can't always count on people not to pass the news on to people you didn't want to know.
You can get all the support you need without the risks of telling everyone at this stage.	

OTHER POINTS TO CONSIDER

- The miscarriage risk is approximately 15% for a first pregnancy and then 19% for a subsequent pregnancy (these figures are based on the period after the woman is likely to know she is pregnant).

- Both prospective parents need to agree on this decision, and stick to it. If you decide not to tell anyone and then one of you can't help giving the news away to their parents, for example, this is likely to cause ructions to say the least (especially when the other set of parents find out that they were the last to know).

- If you're telling only some people and not others, you need to make sure the first lot know they're sworn to secrecy.

- It's worth agreeing a response if anyone guesses and asks you directly. It does happen.

- I may be too late to give you this piece of advice but ... if your friends and family know you're trying for a baby, or perhaps having fertility treatment, they're much more likely to guess or even to know when you get pregnant. If you don't want them to know, don't tell them too much about your attempts to get there.

- Sometimes not everyone will be pleased to hear your news. Whether it's your ex, your infertile sister, or the in-laws who have been harbouring a not-so-secret desire that the two of you will split up, think carefully about how you are going to break the news.

- Remember that some people may be very sensitive about the order you tell people in. If one set of parents finds out that the other knew first, or your brother is on holiday when you break the news and finds out a week after everyone else, you could cause an upset. So think about who you tell when, and how.

- It's worth pointing out that a miscarriage can be almost as upsetting for the prospective father as for his partner. This is further compounded by the fact that, if it happens, it's usually his job to tell everyone the bad news. So both your views on this decision are equally important.

The deadline

About 11½ weeks, presumably.

Worst case scenario

The biggest risk is that you'll tell everyone and then miscarry. It happens and it's not the end of the world, but a miscarriage is much tougher to cope with if everyone knows.

ASK YOURSELF

- How will you feel if you're unlucky enough to have a miscarriage and have already told everyone?
- Do you feel you need support from friends or family before you reach the 13 week stage?
- If you're not going to tell everyone, who's in and who's out?
- How will you tell people?
- What order will you tell them in?
- Is there anyone who needs particularly sensitive handling when you tell them?

2

When to tell the boss

Some people's bosses are also their best mates, and will be among the first to know. But not everyone has that kind of relationship with their employer, and you may fear some kind of reprisal from your boss once they find out you're pregnant. Whether you're right (or they're within their rights) you may worry they'll give the best projects to other people if they think you'll be gone before the end of the project, or will discriminate in other ways against you.

THE FACTS: GIVING NOTICE

You are obliged to tell your employer of your intention to take maternity leave by the end of the 15th week before the week your baby is due.

The options

Another how long is a piece of string question. But basically your options are:

- tell them when you tell other people
- tell them as late as possible (ie up to 26 weeks)

TELL THEM WHEN YOU TELL OTHER PEOPLE

The last section covered when to tell your family and friends that you're pregnant. So this option entails telling your boss at the same time.

Pros	Cons
It makes life a lot easier if you don't have to hide it.	You may fear that your boss will treat you differently knowing you're pregnant.
You can discuss maternity leave options with your boss if you want to, which you may find helpful.	You may feel your boss will put you under pressure to make a decision about maternity leave sooner than you're ready to.

It's easier to avoid heavy lifting and so on at work if the boss knows.	If you miscarry, you may find it particularly hard telling your employer.

TELL THEM AS LATE AS POSSIBLE

Your boss has to find out eventually, but you may want to conceal your pregnancy from them for as long as you can.

Pros	Cons
Your boss can't treat you differently if they don't know you're pregnant.	If friends at work know it may be hard keeping the information from your boss.
You're free to make your own decisions on matters such as maternity leave without any feeling of pressure from your boss.	It can be tricky hiding any morning sickness, avoiding any heavy lifting or working with hazardous substances, and taking time off for scans.
	There comes a point when it will be physically difficult to conceal the pregnancy.

OTHER POINTS TO CONSIDER

- It's much easier organising time off for scans and appointments if your boss knows you're pregnant. (You are entitled to time off for routine antenatal appointments, exercise and antenatal classes, as well as hospital appointments.) If you're lucky you may even have a boss who is flexible about your hours when you're feeling tired or unwell – they may allow you to work from home, or start work later in the mornings.

- Some jobs involve advance planning on a similar scale to pregnancy. If you do project based work, and anything upcoming will partly clash with your maternity leave, it's worth thinking about how to handle this. If your boss knows you'll be on leave, they may not put you on the project in the first place. You might consider this a good thing or a bad thing. If you want to be involved, you might be able to negotiate a compromise that suits both of you, if they know you're pregnant. It depends on your boss, of course.

The deadline

You have to tell your boss by the time you're 26 weeks pregnant.

Worst case scenario

You tell your boss early and they discriminate against you in some way because you're pregnant. This is, of course, illegal – and very few bosses would seriously do this – but it isn't impossible. You could take them to a tribunal of course, but who wants to worry about that when they're coping with a new baby too? Besides, you can't necessarily prove discrimination if they simply allocate to someone else a particular task that didn't officially have your name on it in the first place.

ASK YOURSELF

- How do you feel about your boss knowing you're pregnant?
- Do you think your boss will resent you being pregnant?
- Is your boss likely to be supportive and helpful if they know?
- Are there any major projects coming up at work that might conflict with your maternity leave?

3

When to go on maternity leave

This is such a tricky question, especially if it's your first pregnancy, as you really have no idea how you'll feel after the baby's born. Nevertheless you're expected to give your employer some kind of idea of when you'll be gone, not unreasonably, so they can provide cover. In case you're interested, three quarters of working mothers in the UK take their full paid maternity leave.

THE FACTS: MATERNITY LEAVE

- You're entitled to 39 weeks' maternity leave, usually with maternity pay.

- If, by the beginning of the 14th week before your baby is due, you've been working for your current employer continuously for at least 26 weeks, you can take another 13 weeks' unpaid leave if you wish.

- If you have worked for your current employer continuously for at least a year, you are also entitled to 13 weeks' unpaid parental leave for each child you have. You can take this any time up to your child's fifth birthday, but you are entitled to take it immediately following your maternity leave if you wish.

THE FACTS: GIVING NOTICE

- Your maternity leave cannot start more than 11 weeks before your baby is due.

- You must tell your employer that you intend to take maternity leave by the end of the 15th week before your due date (ie when you're 26 weeks pregnant).

- If you change your mind about when you want the leave to start you must give your employer 28 days' notice (if the baby arrives unexpectedly early you're excused this one).

- The assumption is that you'll take your full maternity entitlement of either 39 weeks or, if you qualify, 52 weeks. If you want to return to work before this time you must give your employer 28 days' notice.

The options

Obviously the options here are almost limitless, but basically the longer you take before the birth, the less time you'll get after it and vice versa. So the three key things you'll want to consider are:

- leaving well before the due date
- staying at work until close to the due date to get longer afterwards
- taking extra unpaid leave beyond your basic nine months after the birth

LEAVING WELL BEFORE THE DUE DATE

This can be popular with women who have an exhausting commute to work. It may also be a good move if you anticipate any health problems ahead of the pregnancy (though unless there's an emergency you'll need 28 days' notice of this).

Pros	Cons
You may be feeling tired and perhaps unwell and you'll appreciate the rest.	You may get bored waiting for the baby to be born.
You have time to get things ready without feeling any pressure to rush.	If most of your friends work you may miss the social support of your work colleagues.
	You'll have to return to work sooner after the birth.

STAYING UNTIL NEAR THE DUE DATE

This certainly keeps you busy, and if you have the energy it's a popular option.

Pros	Cons
You get more time after the birth with your baby before you go back to work.	It can be exhausting, especially if you have a tiring commute.
You don't get time to be bored waiting for the birth.	If the baby is early you may get little or no break before it arrives.

TAKING EXTRA UNPAID LEAVE

At the end of your nine months' leave you can take an additional three months' unpaid leave (and even tack on your three months unpaid parental leave allowance too if you like).

Pros	Cons
You can stay at home with your baby until it is a year old or more.	Additional leave is unpaid so you may struggle financially.
	Some women would happily never go back to work, but others get bored without the mental stimulation of work.

OTHER POINTS TO CONSIDER

- The guidelines set out above are your legal rights. Many employers are sticklers for such things, but not all. It isn't fair to mess your employer about – after all they do need to be able to make sure someone is doing your job in your absence – and it's a rare employer that can afford to pay more than the statutory requirement. However some bosses are pretty flexible when they can be. If they can provide cover fairly easily they may well be flexible about periods of notice, or allow you to work part time in the run up to going on leave.

- It's worth bearing in mind that you may have to start your maternity leave earlier than planned for health reasons – if you're aware of this possibility you'll cope better if it happens. A number of conditions in later pregnancy such as hypertensive disorders or SPD (symphysis pubis dysfunction – which can lead to considerable pain in the hip joints especially) can mean you need to leave work early.

- Many women choose to take maternity leave and then decide they don't want to return to work yet. In that case you can hand in your notice and not return to work at all until you want or need to.

- Depending on your contract of employment, you may be able to extend your maternity leave with holiday allowance. Many women save up holiday to take before the baby is born so that they can leave, say, a month before it's born but their maternity leave starts later. With some contracts you may also be able to take next year's holiday allowance starting on the day you officially return to work, so you actually return a few weeks later.

- If you plan to breastfeed this may influence your decision about when to return to work. You can express milk after you have gone back to work, but some women don't enjoy this option and prefer either to stop breastfeeding or to take longer maternity leave. It's unlikely to be the only factor in making the decision on when to return, but you may want to take it into account.

- Fathers (or the mother's partner) are entitled to take up to six months' paternity leave during the baby's first year. However only one of you can be paid at a time. The father only qualifies for statutory paternity pay if the mother has returned to work and is therefore not drawing her entitled pay – in other words only up to nine months after the start of her maternity leave. And she must have taken at least six months' leave, so there's only a three month window during which the father can receive paternity pay. (More on paternity pay in chapter 4.)

The deadline

You have to tell your employer when you intend to go on maternity leave by the time you are 26 weeks pregnant. You can change your mind after this but you must give 28 days' notice. You don't have to make a decision about when to return to work until your baby is several months old.

Worst case scenario

Most mothers would tell you that the worst thing is having to leave the baby to go back to work sooner than you feel ready to. Mind you, unless you can afford not to go back to work at all you'll have to face this sometime, and it's always tough. You may never feel ready.

ASK YOURSELF

- How much maternity leave can you afford to take?

- Are you likely to miss work if you take a long break? Are you the type to get bored with only a baby for company or will you enjoy it?

- How flexible/amenable is your boss?

- Are you both planning to take leave? How will you distribute the leave between the two of you?

- Do you have any holiday entitlement you can use to extend your leave?

- Are you planning to breastfeed, and for how long?

4

What paternity leave to take

Fathers take their relationships with their babies far more seriously than they did in our parents' generation, and certainly all the research shows that children benefit from a close relationship with their father. And there's no doubt that (breastfeeding apart) fathers are equally capable of caring for and bonding with a baby.

THE FACTS: PATERNITY LEAVE

- You are entitled to up to two weeks' paid leave, assuming you qualify (you must have a responsibility for the child, be its natural father or its mother's partner, and have been working continuously for a minimum period for the same employer).

- You will receive statutory paternity pay for this leave.

- You can also take up to six months' leave during the first year of the baby's life. This will be unpaid *unless* (concentrate now, this can be confusing) the baby's mother has returned to work before using up her full maternity pay entitlement (which she will do nine months after going on maternity leave). *And* she must have taken at least six months' maternity leave. So only one of you at a time can claim maternity/paternity pay, and you can't claim it for more than three of your possible six months.

THE FACTS: GIVING NOTICE

- You must tell your employer that you plan to take paternity leave before your partner is 26 weeks pregnant (unless this isn't possible for some reason). You must also let them know when the baby is due, and how much leave you intend to take.

- You must give your employer at least 28 days' notice of when you want your leave to start. If you give them more warning than this, you are allowed to change your mind up to this point. (If the baby is premature you'll be let off the 28 day thing.)

The options

You have the following choices:

- take no paternity leave at all
- take up to two weeks' paid leave
- take up to six months' unpaid leave (or paid leave in place of your partner's leave, if you qualify)

TAKE NO PATERNITY LEAVE

There's no legal requirement to take any time off at all when your baby is born.

Pros	Cons
You avoid most of the hard work.	You miss out on the chance to bond with your baby, which almost all fathers will tell you is worth the hard work.
You don't have to take a pay cut.	Unless you've got a damn good reason for it, your partner will almost certainly hate you.
You may avoid spending several weeks as a zombie.	Unless you get an unrealistically amenable baby, or give your partner no support whatever, you'll spend the first couple of weeks functioning well below par at work due to exhaustion.

TAKE UP TO TWO WEEKS' PAID LEAVE

This is a popular option, and enables you to concentrate on the family at the most critical time, immediately following the birth.

Pros	Cons
Your partner will really appreciate you being there, and you'll be able to help fully without worrying about being unfit for work due to exhaustion.	Statutory paternity pay is lower than your normal salary.
You'll get a chance to bond properly with your baby at the most critical time.	Going back to work after two weeks will probably feel far too soon, at least at the time.

TAKE UP TO SIX MONTHS' UNPAID LEAVE

Obviously you don't have to take the full six months if you don't want to. You might want to take just a month or two.

Pros	Cons
You get to spend more time with your new baby.	You'll suffer a significant drop in earnings if you take the full entitlement.
You ease the load on your partner for longer.	You may find you miss work if you spend too long away.
You get a chance to sample full time parenting, if this is an option you're considering.	

OTHER POINTS TO CONSIDER

- You may well be able to extend your paternity leave by judicious use of holiday entitlement.

- You can elect to start your paternity leave either on the day the baby is born, or after it's born (but you must finish the leave no more than 56 days after the birth), or anytime from the first day of the week in which the baby is due. Be warned: if you start your leave on or around the date the baby is due *and then it's late* it is theoretically quite possible to find that you have no leave left by the time the baby actually arrives.

- Sleep deprivation is perhaps the toughest part of coping with a new baby. You can share the burden with your partner far more easily if you're not working. If you have to leave the house early each morning you'll need at least a half decent night's sleep, which puts the burden back on your partner. This is perhaps the biggest consideration when deciding how much leave to take – not helped by the fact that you have no idea how well the baby will sleep. Some sleep all night and some are awake all night – and others cover all points in between – and you've no idea which you're going to get.

- The sleep deprivation problem improves significantly by around six weeks (though it may still be bad), and by about three months you should manage a passable night's sleep more often than not. You won't catch up, and you'll still feel knackered (for most of the next 18 years actually) but you'll be able to cope. All babies are different, blah blah blah, but this is about as bad as it gets, and this information may help you plan how much paternity leave you want to take.

- If you already have another child (who is still young) it can be extremely hard for your partner to look after it properly, especially if she is breastfeeding. Many fathers on paternity leave concentrate on giving the older child or children care, attention and continuity while the mother is looking after the baby.

- If you are expecting twins (or more) be warned that everyone says that these fathers always get really involved – because there's no choice. You can virtually guarantee that unless your partner has a lot of other help, she will struggle desperately if you don't take time out to support her. How much time you will need varies, of course, according to circumstances, but you'd do well to think in terms of taking your full fortnight's paid leave and then either some unpaid leave or holiday for the next couple of weeks or more.

- Remember that by law you are now allowed to ask your employer for flexible working if you have a child under six (or a disabled child under 18). This includes part time working, working from home, job sharing, and working only during term time. By law your employer must give your request 'serious consideration', and can refuse only for 'sound business reasons' such as extra costs.

- In families where the woman earns more than the man, it's not unusual for the mother to return to work (eventually) while the father takes on the full time parent job. If you're considering this option, a period of unpaid paternity leave (or paid if your partner returns to work between six and nine months) can help you decide whether this works for you both. (I'd also recommend the book *Full Time Father* by Richard Hallows, published by White Ladder.)

The deadline

You need to make a decision on whether to take leave by the time your partner is 26 weeks pregnant. You have until about 36 weeks to decide when you're going to take it.

Worst case scenario

The worst case scenario would probably be if you took little or no leave and then saw your partner struggling to cope. Of course you have no idea in advance whether your partner will struggle, as it has a great deal to do with the baby itself, how well it sleeps, whether it cries a lot and so on. However even in this case you might well be able to take holiday entitlement in order to help out.

ASK YOURSELF

- How much leave can you afford to take?

- Do you have holiday entitlement you could use?

- How much support and help will your partner have from elsewhere?

- How do you *both* feel about how much leave you should take?

- How flexible/amenable is your employer?

- Do you already have any other young children? What care arrangements do you have for them in the first few weeks of the new baby?

- How involved a father would you ideally want to be?

- Are you expecting twins or triplets?

- Is being a full time father an option you want to keep open?

- Would you consider flexible working after your paternity leave?

5

How much to eat during pregnancy

Obviously you're going to put on weight during the pregnancy. Presumably you want to put on as much weight as the baby needs you too, and then afterwards return to the weight you were before you got pregnant or thereabouts. The tricky bit is knowing how to do this. The medical professionals will tell you (irritatingly but quite rightly) that everyone is different and there are no hard and fast rules about how much weight you should gain, or at what stage in the pregnancy. Accurate, but not helpful…

The options

Your choices are to:

- eat anything
- be reasonably careful about what you eat but don't think about it too much
- diet while pregnant

EAT WHATEVER AND WORRY ABOUT IT LATER

This is clearly the most appealing option. If you're hungry, you eat. Of course you may find yourself putting on weight rather quickly but hey, you've got the rest of your life to lose it again.

Pros	Cons
It's more fun.	You could end up a lot heavier after the pregnancy than you were before.
If you're not limiting your diet it's easier to get all the energy and nutrients you need.	There is an increased risk of pregnancy diabetes, though your overall weight and other factors will be relevant. It's a risk, not a certainty, but one to consider if the weight starts piling on.
You'll get tired during pregnancy whatever you eat, but this way you'll be getting enough energy not to exacerbate the tiredness.	

BE CAREFUL BUT DON'T THINK ABOUT IT TOO MUCH

This is the laid back option. You avoid obviously fattening foods but you don't stand on the scales every day or count calories. The idea here is that you can be pretty confident of not putting on too much weight as you're not eating anything particularly fattening.

Pros	Cons
It's easy, although not quite as much fun as the previous option.	It's quite hard to judge how much weight you're gaining.
This approach probably gives you the best chance of eating a diet that is healthy for you and the baby, as you'll presumably be monitoring the quality of what you eat.	You run the risk of finding at the end of the pregnancy that you're left with more extra weight than you'd anticipated.

DIET SO YOU DON'T PUT ON EXCESS WEIGHT

This approach involves counting calories or restricting food groups in order to make sure that you don't put on more weight than you need. I should add that you'll struggle to find any health professional who would endorse actively dieting during pregnancy as there are health risks for both you and the baby. The only partial exception is that if you are already obese you would be wise to be careful about what you eat.

Pros	Cons
You should manage to avoid putting on excess weight.	The baby's birth weight may suffer, and its overall health can also be damaged if you avoid certain food groups.
It's likely that you'll avoid unhealthy foods on this kind of regime.	Your body needs extra nutrients and energy to get you through pregnancy, so you may suffer health problems.
	You may get very tired if you're not getting all the extra energy your body needs.

HOW MUCH WEIGHT SHOULD YOU GAIN?

Wouldn't it be nice if there were a simple answer to this question? It's the boring old, unhelpful 'everyone's different' thing again. However, I'll try to give you broad indications at least, as long as you promise not to hold me to it:

- Most women (who don't gain excess weight) add an average of 26½lbs (12kg) during their pregnancy. This is made up of the weight of the baby itself, the amniotic fluid, the placenta and so on, and most of it will go within a couple of weeks of the birth.

- Typical weight gain in the first 20 weeks is around 5lbs.

- Typical weight gain in the second 20 weeks is around 1lb a week.

- Women who are obese may gain less than this, and women who are thinner to start with may gain weight more rapidly.

OTHER POINTS TO CONSIDER

- Most of us have a pretty canny idea of how easy we find it to lose weight. If everyone in your family looks like a stick and weight falls off you as you blink, you probably don't need to fret too much about what you eat. Then again, if everyone in your family looks like a football and just looking at food makes you fat, there's a fair chance that you'll end up overweight if you're not careful.

- What you eat is far more important than how much you eat. I haven't got room to write a complete book here on healthy eating in pregnancy, but you can go and buy one. The gist is obvious though, as far as weight is concerned: avoid high fat, high sugar, processed foods and the like, and eat lots of healthy fruit and vegetables, and lean meat and fish, and extra dairy products for calcium.

- A few women have the opposite problem from the normal one: they feel so sick that they struggle to eat enough. In this case it's more important than ever that you try to make sure that everything you *do* eat is good for you and the baby. If this persists for any length of time you'll need to talk to your doctor or midwife for advice. (I should warn you that although this is very unpleasant, there's no point looking for sympathy from any of your overweight friends. If you need a shoulder to cry on, find a bony one.)

- The older you are, the harder it will be to lose any excess weight afterwards, particularly once you get past about 30.

- Breastfeeding should help you to lose extra weight since the body is designed to build up energy (in the form of fat) during pregnancy, to use during breastfeeding. If you don't breastfeed you won't use this up naturally and will have to find some other method if you want to lose it. Don't, however, rely on losing lots of extra weight by breastfeeding as it doesn't always happen.

- If you are expecting twins or more, you are twice as likely to suffer anaemia so it's a good idea to eat plenty of iron- and folate-rich foods.

The deadline

You need to make this decision in the first few weeks. Some women start putting on weight within the first couple of months, and your appetite can change that early on. Of course, you might be one of those women whose pregnancy hardly shows for months, but it's worth thinking about this before your body responds to being pregnant. Having said that, this is a decision you can revise as you go through the pregnancy. But you'll find it helpful to have a general policy from the early weeks.

Worst case scenario

The worst case of all is that you diet too much and the baby's health is adversely affected. Low birthweight babies are more likely to suffer disabilities and general health problems, and are at 40 times greater risk of death during the first month of life.

You could end up far heavier than you started (potentially stones not pounds). There is also an increased risk of both gestational diabetes and pregnancy-induced hypertension, both of which increase the likelihood of having to have a caesarean section. Being obese or gaining excessive weight also raises the risk of urinary tract infections, difficulty determining the foetal position, postpartum haemorrhage and thrombophlebitis (a condition which can lead to thrombosis).

- How easy do you find it to lose weight?

- Are you prone to being underweight?

- How healthy is your diet?

- How have other close women relatives (especially your mother and any sisters) responded to being pregnant? Is there a family tendency to gain too much or too little weight, or to have trouble losing it afterwards?

- Do you or the baby have any conditions which might impinge on this? Are you diabetic? Is there any other reason why your baby is at high risk of having a low birth weight?

6

What should and shouldn't you eat?

If you go looking for it, there is a wealth of information out there in books, magazines and the internet on what you should and shouldn't be eating during pregnancy. Generally speaking, a healthy diet rich in nutrients and low in sugar and fat will suffice, but you'd be surprised how often somebody will offer you advice on what you should be avoiding. As medical advice changes practically daily, I've set out what seems to be the most common-sense approach to eating high-risk foods during pregnancy so you can feel free to make the right decisions for you.

The options

There are probably three ways for you to go about making choices about high-risk foods:

- avoid anything considered high-risk by the medical industry
- eat everything you want to
- choose your eating habits carefully and base decisions around individual food items only

AVOID ANYTHING CONSIDERED TO BE HIGH-RISK

For some women, this is the safest and only option, but in practical terms it can be incredibly difficult to abide by. A lot of the items on the high-risk list are to be avoided during your first trimester, but if you're choosing not to tell people you're pregnant until after this period you may have to make some difficult choices when out in public.

Pros	Cons
Any possible risk to your baby from food-borne illnesses is reduced.	Making choices in your first trimester can be difficult if you're not going public.
You'll have peace of mind and no reason to feel guilty.	You don't get to eat everything you want to, even if you're craving it.

You may feel healthier if your diet is improved by cutting out alcohol and caffeine, for example.	You may resent your pregnancy for determining your choices.

EAT EVERYTHING YOU WANT TO

Eating everything you want to during your pregnancy does carry some risks, but it also means you don't have to change much about your lifestyle in the early stages. If you have been pregnant before and were fine, you may also be fine this time around, no matter what diet you follow.

Pros	Cons
You can eat whatever and whenever you want to.	You can potentially put your baby at risk from food-borne illnesses.
You won't have to explain to other people why you no longer eat brie if you don't want to.	You may feel guilty and/or unhealthy.
Your regular diet doesn't have to change much, which means it won't cost more and will be easier to manage.	

CHOOSE FOOD CAREFULLY

This seems to be the most common-sense approach to high-risk foods. Obviously you don't want to put your unborn child at any kind of risk, but if you also know that there is no history of allergic reactions in your family to peanuts, why shouldn't you indulge every so often? As with many things, the more you consume of a food, the higher the risk there will be something wrong with it, so eating a small amount of what you really enjoy, or deciding to cut it out completely if the risk is too high for your conscience, may make you the happiest in the long run.

All the advice offered by the NHS on what foods to avoid is based on current scientific evidence. However some of it is exceedingly cautious. There is plenty of information if you want to look for it, in books and on the internet, about the facts and figures behind this advice. This can help you to make informed decisions for yourself.

Pros	Cons
Deciding to indulge or to decline is a personal choice, leaving you in control of your diet.	You might still have to answer awkward questions early on in your pregnancy.
You may be happiest knowing you're making decisions based upon careful thought.	As all these foods carry a risk, if you choose to eat any of them you may put your baby at risk.
If you do choose to not eat the most high-risk foods, you are still protecting your child.	

OTHER POINTS TO CONSIDER

- Clearly there are reasons why researchers have defined some foods as high-risk and you may well want to consider these carefully before consuming them.

- Some styles of cooking require more high-risk foods than others, such as the heavy use of fish and peanuts in Oriental dishes.

- A lot of the risks are increased by the amount you consume, so eating very small quantities of your favourite item when you're really craving it is far less risky overall than eating it frequently.

- There are some very good substitutes out there if you really crave something. Vegetarian deli meats or decaffeinated coffee will probably do just as well for the next few months.

Deadline

For some high-risk items on this list your decision needs to be made immediately, such as with consuming alcohol or caffeine. For others it can be delayed until you come across them, as unless you really like eating shark, chances are it's not something you eat every day anyway.

Worst case scenario

The very worst case scenario here is that by eating a high-risk food you pass on something unpleasant to your unborn baby, resulting in a possible birth defect, miscarriage or even stillbirth.

ASK YOURSELF

- Am I happy to tell people I'm pregnant straightaway if they ask questions about why I'm no longer drinking my usual rum and coke? How do I feel about people knowing that early on?

- How much of a risk am I prepared to put both myself and my baby at?

- How many of these high-risk items do I actually eat?

- Am I happy to give up my favourite cheeses for nine months?

- Are there foods I'll struggle to manage without? Could I work out a system or make substitutions instead?

- Am I prepared to change my cooking style for the duration of the pregnancy?

FOODS YOU'RE ADVISED TO STAY AWAY FROM

Seafood

Consuming seafood is generally considered safe during pregnancy, with the exception of swordfish, shark, king mackerel and tilefish (blanquillo). These bigger fish can contain large amounts of mercury, which may damage a developing embryo's nervous system. Other types of seafood, such as shrimp, canned tuna, salmon, pollock and catfish are actually encouraged, as the benefits of omega-3 fats for embryos far outweigh any potential risks from mercury. Fish should always be cooked properly, so oysters and mussels should not be eaten raw, and some researchers even go as far as to suggest avoiding smoked fish as this cannot be guaranteed to have been cooked through correctly.

Undercooked meat and poultry

It's wise to avoid undercooked meat and poultry even when you're not pregnant, but women should pay particular attention when they are. Medical professionals recommend cooking steaks and hamburgers to a minimum of medium and avoiding excessive amounts of deli-style meats, such as ham and sandwich turkey as they can potentially carry dangerous bacteria.

Pâté

This carries a risk of listeria so the official advice is not to eat it.

Liver and vitamin A supplements

The argument against liver is that it contains high levels of vitamin A, and there is a small risk that excessive quantities of this can harm your baby.

Raw and partially cooked eggs

There is a slight risk of salmonella if you eat eggs which aren't fully cooked through, so the advice is that they should be cooked until both the yolk and white are solid. Most brands of mayonnaise, ice creams, dressings and so on will be made with pasteurised eggs so they're fine. However home made versions may contain uncooked egg in which case the advice is not to eat them.

Dairy products containing unpasteurised milk

The main products to contain unpasteurised milk tend to be soft cheeses, so unless a packet of your favourite smelly cheese is clearly labelled as made with pasteurised milk, it's advised you avoid Brie, feta, Camembert, blue cheeses and some soft Spanish and Mexican cheeses. These cheeses can contain nasty bacteria, which you obviously don't want to pass on to your little one.

Peanuts and honey

If you have a family history of peanut allergies, eczema, asthma or hay fever, some doctors may recommend you do not consume peanuts while pregnant in order to reduce the risk of passing allergies on to your unborn child. However, studies have not been conclusive and the only correlation at present seems to be that the more you eat, the higher the risk. Honey is generally not pasteurised and can potentially contain harmful spores which lead to the growth of nasty bacteria in the gut, but while this is obviously a very big no-no for infants under one year old, it's generally considered safe for pregnant women.

Caffeine

For a lot of women, caffeine is probably the hardest item on this list to learn to live without while you're pregnant. Caffeine increases yours and your baby's heart rate and some studies have shown it can lead to low birth weight infants or miscarriage and stillbirth. Experts advise completely cutting out caffeine during your first trimester and only consuming a maximum of 200mg per day after that, which is the equivalent to around two cups of coffee, tea or cola. Also worth remembering is that caffeine is also found in chocolate, more's the pity.

Herbal teas

Herbal teas can be a lifesaver for some women, particularly those suffering from bad morning sickness, but the latest advice is that as there isn't enough research into the effects of certain herbs on the body, excessive amounts of these types of tea should be avoided. Red raspberry leaf tea, for example, has been found to induce contractions and even full-blown labour if drunk in large quantities. While this might be quite useful if you're anxiously awaiting your new baby past 40 weeks, it's probably wise not to drink it before then.

Alcohol

There is conflicting evidence on the consumption of alcohol during pregnancy, but the general consensus is that as there is no definitive 'safe' amount, all alcohol should be cut out completely. Obviously a small sip of wine at a party will not result in a poorly baby with foetal alcohol syndrome, but as the effects of even small regular quantities are not yet known, experts advise laying off the booze entirely.

7

Will you go to antenatal classes?

Most women attend some kind of antenatal class. Many swear by them while others suspect they're a waste of time. In the end it's down to your own personal confidence and preferences. So you need to know what they actually involve, and what you might gain by going.

The options

You have two options essentially:

- go to antenatal classes
- don't bother with them

GO TO ANTENATAL CLASSES

Most women go for this option, and to be honest I've met the odd woman who felt that the course they attended wasn't the best, but I've never met anyone who regretted going. It's usual to go only for your first pregnancy.

Pros	Cons
Your confidence will be boosted by feeling you have some knowledge to support you.	It's a commitment in time, though your employer should give you time off if you're still at work.
You'll learn useful skills to help you through labour.	If the course isn't the right one for you, you may not feel at ease.
You'll make lots of new friends going through the same thing you are.	
You may find it easier to make decisions under stress if the birth doesn't go exactly to plan.	

DON'T BOTHER WITH THEM

A lot of women who don't go to classes have some reason for feeling they don't need them. Perhaps they have experience of newborns already, or have a great deal of support lined up.

Pros	Cons
You don't have to drag yourself off to classes when you're heavily pregnant.	You'll miss out on a lot of information that you might have found useful.
If you're not a 'group' kind of person you may be happier not going.	You'll miss the opportunity to make friends.
	If you don't have a textbook labour, you may find it harder to make the best choices, especially if your knowledge is limited.

OTHER POINTS TO CONSIDER

● Antenatal classes focus largely, though not exclusively, on childbirth. You should learn to recognise the start of labour, how to breathe once contractions start, what pain relief is available and so on. You'll also learn how to stay fit and comfortable during pregnancy, especially how to protect your back and your body.

● Some classes prepare you better than others for coping with a non-standard labour. If you've been prepared for a textbook delivery and then hit problems it can be a shock and hard to cope. So it's worth checking the class you sign up for prepares you for the options if things don't go to plan.

- Many women say later, with hindsight, that the best thing about antenatal classes was the longstanding friendships they made, and the ready made set of friends for their new baby to grow up with.

- There are lots of different classes available. Broadly speaking there are free classes, run by local hospitals or midwives, and private classes run by organisations such as the NCT (National Childbirth Trust), or the Active Birth Centre, which you'll probably have to pay for. You can always go to more than one lot of classes if you want to.

- It's a good move to ask friends with young children to recommend a local class to you. Different classes suit different people so do as much research as you can. Although it's probably wise to avoid classes where the teacher has a real crusade for or against any particular kind of birth, you'll find that most classes have some kind of bias, albeit an understandable one. For example, a hospital class is likely to favour a hospital birth, and almost all classes will encourage you to breastfeed, some more forcefully than others. Of course they're quite right that breast milk is best for your baby, but it's your choice how you feed and some classes may put you under more pressure than others.

- If you go for a private class, make sure the teacher has been properly trained.

- Some classes are for mothers only, some expect partners to attend too, some are open about whether or not you both go. You'll find that some men report finding antenatal classes very helpful and involving, while other men will tell you they felt extremely uncomfortable and excluded. It depends largely on the class, so if you both want to go it's a good idea to research this carefully, asking as many men as you reasonably can for recommendations.

● In some rural areas courses may be held quite far apart, so check when they run to make sure you don't miss the window.

The deadline

Most classes run for six to eight week courses towards the end of pregnancy. They can get booked up early though so you need to decide fairly early on in order to be sure of getting a place. In some parts of the country you may need to book as early as 12 weeks. There'll almost certainly be more than one course in your area so if you miss out on one you can book another.

Worst case scenario

The worst that can happen is that you find the birth more uncomfortable because you missed out on learning about relaxation techniques and the options open to you. So although the benefits may be considerable, missing out on antenatal classes isn't a catastrophe.

ASK YOURSELF

● Do you feel you could learn something useful from antenatal classes?

● Are you the kind of person who would relish the opportunity to make new friends?

● Can you afford to pay?

● Do you both want to attend?

8

Will you need help?

Lots of parents look after their children with no outside help at all. However, it depends very much on your circumstances. If you both work, if you're a single parent, if you're expecting twins or more, if you're disabled or have other responsibilities such as elderly relatives to care for – or if you just fancy an easy ride (and who doesn't?) – you may well want to organise some kind of help looking after the baby. I'm not going to go into childcare once your child is older; I'll concentrate on the sort of thing you might well be planning for while you're still pregnant.

The options

Broadly speaking the options range from having no help to having permanent live-in help, and all points in between. The basic options are:

- look after the baby yourselves
- get help from a relative
- pay for part time help
- pay for full time, live-in help

Cost is obviously a factor, and what you want isn't necessarily going to be what you can afford, so you'll need to investigate ahead of time what you'll have to pay for help if you decide to go for that option.

LOOK AFTER THE BABY YOURSELVES

Obviously this has worked for centuries, and still works for many people. However times have changed, and it doesn't work for everyone now. Bear in mind that people used to live in close-knit social groups. Many still do, and if your mum is down the road and your sister-in-law's round the corner they will probably help out when you need it.

However, if you live some distance from your family and close friends you can't rely on the same level of day-to-day support. That means that if the baby screams for hours when you've had no sleep, there's no one to take it off your hands so you can have a break. If you come down with some ghastly bug, you still have to keep changing the nappies between bouts of vomiting (OK, let's not go there until we have to).

Another point to make here is that many couples now have quite flexible work arrangements and can work from home at least some of the time. I don't want to patronise in any way, but it needs to be said: almost every couple I know in this situation has said during the pregnancy that one of them will look after the baby while they're working at home. And every one has discovered in the event that it isn't possible (myself included). You cannot work and look after a baby, and it's rash to plan on the assumption that you can. Occasionally you may get five minutes' work done, or even half an hour on a really good day, but often you manage none at all.

Pros	Cons
You feel as involved as possible with your baby, and not prone to the guilt that so notoriously besets many parents who leave the baby with someone else.	You can't work full time and look after a baby, so if you both want to go back to work this option is not going to be feasible.
It's the cheapest option.	It can be exhausting, though this is reduced if there are two parents sharing the babycare.

GET HELP FROM A RELATIVE

I'm not talking about the occasional phone call to say, 'Help! The washing machine's leaking, the freezer's defrosted itself, the baby has pooed so much there are no clean clothes left, and I haven't slept for 17 days 21 hours and eight minutes.' I'm talking about an arrangement where your relative looks after the baby two mornings a week while you shop or work (or sleep), or has them every Friday, or whatever.

Of course, you need to have a suitable and willing volunteer, with the time available, for this to be an option for you.

Pros	Cons
You have help from someone who is part of the baby's family and whom you can trust (presumably, or you wouldn't be asking them).	If you don't agree with their style you can't sack them without causing family tension. For some people this option is brilliant, but for some it can cause huge stress.
It's generally free, or at least very inexpensive.	If you're not paying, you may feel very uncomfortable asking them to put in extra time.
If your relative doesn't work, they are likely to be more flexible about hours than most paid helpers would be.	

PAY FOR SOME KIND OF PART-TIME HELP

There are lots of variations here in terms of hours, duties and so on. But broadly speaking you pay someone for a fixed number of hours to help you in whatever way you've agreed. So they may come to your house just to look after the baby, or they may help with other chores to free you up to deal with the baby. Or you may leave the baby with them at their house once you go back to work.

When my first son was born, we made the classic mistake (see above) of thinking we could both work from home and look after him between us. When he was two months old I started working again, and we realised this was a completely daft idea and we needed help. So we found someone who lived nearby and came to the house for two or three hours a day to look after him. If he slept (which I don't actually remember him doing), or when I was feeding him, she cleared the kitchen, put a wash through the machine and tidied up.

Now, over nine years (and two more babies) later, she is still with us and as fabulous and invaluable as ever. If you can find the right person this really is a good system, but it does depend heavily on the helper fitting into the family well.

Pros	Cons
You have regular help at the time – and in the way – you want it.	It will cost you, obviously, though how much depends on how many hours you want them to work.
If there are problems, or if your helper doesn't work out, it's much easier to resolve professionally than the family angst of having to tell, say, your mother-in-law that you don't approve of her methods of getting the baby to sleep.	If they're off sick you can be really stuffed, especially if you have work to go to.
	They may not be flexible if you want them to do extra hours for some reason, and this can leave you in the lurch.

HAVE FULL-TIME, LIVE-IN HELP

This is clearly the most expensive option, but also the most relaxing. Whether you go for an au pair or a trained nanny, a live-in helper is always there to help. You need to be very clear before they start exactly what help you're asking for. A nanny may not be happy to undertake, say, cleaning duties, although they should be happy to do anything relating to the baby such as tidying the playroom or sterilising bottles. But do you want them to wash reusable nappies? Cook and prepare baby food? Get up at 3am for the baby? Make sure you have all these details established in advance.

Pros	Cons
You get maximum help this way.	The most expensive choice, obviously.
You have a professional relationship so sorting out problems is easier than with a helper who is also part of your family.	They will need time off. It's a tough job, and they are unlikely to be flexible about working extra hours.
	Some people feel uncomfortable having someone else living in the house permanently.

OTHER POINTS TO CONSIDER

- Your budget is a key part of the equation. You need to be sure you can afford whatever option you choose to take. It's much easier to start with help for just a couple of hours a day and then build up once you're confident the money will stretch. Cutting down your helper's hours if you find you're overstretched means upping yours. However much you love your baby, this will be exhausting and far more stressful. I won't witter on about the huge cost of having a baby because you'll have heard it all before, but do be realistic about your budget.

- If you're thinking of asking for help from one of your parents, consider what their other time commitments are. They will have less energy than they did when their own babies were born, and they may have a job or a very busy life already. However much they love their new grandchild, they may feel that this is a time of life to be extending their freedom rather than their commitments. Some grandparents want nothing more than to be involved on a daily basis with the new baby, but many are reluctant to make such a commitment. So it might be wise not to ask unless you're prepared for them to say no without any ill feeling.

- Everyone has a different view of how to bring up a baby (and actually, most of them are just as good as the next). Think about your views and how they'll fit with your helper's. If you're paying them, you're in charge, but if they're family it's trickier. If you're open to the advice of your parents' generation you may well be very happy having them care for your baby. But if you feel strongly that demand feeding is best, and your mother is equally adamant that babies should be fed once every four hours no matter how much they cry, you might want to think through the potential stress of asking her to look after the baby twice a week.

- If you decide to pay for outside help, remember to check the credentials and references of anyone you're considering thoroughly. Horror stories are incredibly rare, but they do occasionally happen and as it's one of the most crucial decisions you'll make, it's much better to give yourself peace of mind.

The deadline

You don't need to sort this out until the baby is born, but finding the right person (depending on the option you go for) can be difficult so it's worth planning ahead. Obviously if it all goes wrong once the baby arrives you can change the arrangements, but this can be stressful so best to avoid it if you can.

Worst case scenario

The worst scenario is when families fall out. You can change arrangements with childminders and nannies, and you can organise help when you'd thought you'd manage without. It's not ideal because you may be under pressure, but it's manageable.

However, if a close relative looks after the baby and it doesn't work out, there's a risk that you might do lasting damage to your relationship. I don't want to deter you if this is best for you, because it does work extremely well for many families, but you need to give this option the most thought because the most is at stake.

ASK YOURSELF

- Do you want, or feel you'll need, extra help?

- Are you planning to go back to work?

- How much can you afford to pay for help?

- How many hours of help do you think you'll need?

- What sort of help will you want? You might want to pay someone to look after the house so you can concentrate on the baby full time, or you might want help with the baby.

- Are you likely to need a helper whose hours can be flexible?

- Do you have any relatives who would be able to help? And willing?

- Do you think there would be stressful friction with them if they were around a lot and responsible for your baby for several hours a week? If not, does your partner agree with you about this?

- If you're considering live-in help, how would you feel about having someone else in the house permanently?

part two

Decisions about your home

9

Where will the baby sleep?

Obviously the baby will be with you most of the time: in the kitchen, in the living room, at the shops and so on. But it helps to have a kind of base camp where the baby sleeps. So the critical question is where will it sleep (you hope) at night?

A word about 'cot death'

Probably one of the biggest concerns for parents when it comes to anything to do with your baby's sleep, including where they should spend the night, is SIDS (Sudden Infant Death Syndrome). To put the risk in perspective, bear in mind that SIDS is not as common as many parents fear. Somewhere slightly over 300 babies a year die of SIDS; in 2004 this amounted to one in every 2,325 babies. Just under 90% of these are under six months old. Your baby is not at high risk so long as:

- it isn't premature

- it isn't low birthweight

- it doesn't have a previous sibling who died of SIDS

- it doesn't have a mother who smokes or takes drugs

- it doesn't have a mother who was under 20 for her first pregnancy

- it doesn't live in a smoky environment

- it hasn't had a life-threatening episode, especially one connected with breathing problems

- you follow the standard guidelines, putting the baby down to sleep on its back, feet near the foot of the cot so it can't wriggle down under the covers, and making sure it doesn't overheat. Don't put pillows or fluffy toys in with it during the first few months.

Nevertheless, you may still feel that minimising the risk of SIDS is one of the biggest factors in deciding where your baby will sleep.

Bear in mind here that no decision is irreversible, so there's no need to get too stressed about this one. In fact, any option apart from its own room *should* be only temporary. You don't want it in bed with you up until it reaches its teens. However, you'd obviously rather make the right decision first time and save the disruption of having to change a system that doesn't work.

The options

The generally accepted options are:

- in its own room
- in a cot or crib in your room
- in your bed with you

IN ITS OWN ROOM

This is theoretically the most peaceful option, though if you're a worrier you may not find it very relaxing. It does prevent your own bedroom turning into a mess of spare nappies, clothes, blankets, wipes and the rest of it, which for some people means their bedroom can function as a kind of haven, which it certainly isn't if the baby is in there with you. Here are the main pros and cons.

Pros	Cons
It saves having to move the baby later.	It's further to go in the night to feed the baby.
Being dedicated to the baby there's probably more room for all the inexplicable gubbins that babies like to surround themselves with.	You may worry more if you can't see it breathing.
It means your bedroom is peaceful, when you get to spend any time there.	The incidence of SIDS is higher in babies who sleep alone than in those who share a room with their mother (though keep this in perspective if your baby is not otherwise high risk).
It means you don't have to worry about waking the baby every time you roll over or your partner snores.	Babies who sleep alone spend less time asleep than those who sleep in close proximity to their mother (or main care giver).
It means that one of you can sleep undisturbed while the other deals with the baby in the night.	

IN A COT/CRIB IN YOUR ROOM

If you go for this option, you can put the baby anywhere from the furthest corner of the room to right next to your bed where you can reach out and touch it (always a slightly fraught exercise in the dark as your hand might encounter interesting leakages of baby excreta before settling on the baby itself). Evidence shows that the safest thing for your baby (and frankly the most convenient for you) is for the baby to be within arm's reach. Here are some pros and cons.

Pros	Cons
The Foundation for the Study of Infant Deaths recommends that the safest place for a baby to sleep is in a cot beside its parents' bed for the first six months.	Eventually you'll have to move the baby to its own room which can take some adjustment – from both (or all) of you.
You don't have to get out of bed in the night for a breastfeed (though if you bottle feed you may have to go to the kitchen to warm the bottle).	Your bedroom will have to accommodate all the baby bedtime junk, from changing mats to spare clothes.
You can keep a careful watch over the baby through the night.	If the baby is a light sleeper you may occasionally wake it if you are noisy in the night.
	Unless you sleep very deeply, you may be disturbed when your partner is dealing with the baby in the night.
	Once you're in a fit state to resume your sex life, you might find the presence of the baby cramps your style (some couples hate it, others aren't bothered).

IN YOUR BED WITH YOU

This is the closest and most comforting position of all in the view of many parents. On the other hand, some research shows that it is the highest risk option for SIDS (Sudden Infant Death Syndrome). Around 135 of the 300+ SIDS deaths a year in the UK are of babies who shared beds with their parents. Also, if you think your partner steals all the quilt/occupies over half the mattress you'd be amazed how much of a bed can be taken over by a very small baby that can't even roll over yet.

On the other hand, there is also research to show that if your baby is low risk for SIDS, neither of you smokes or drinks, and you are breastfeeding, bedsharing with your baby is as safe as having it next to you in a cot or crib. It is important that you still make sure the baby sleeps on its back, you keep pillows and quilts well away from it, and you sleep in a position that protects it (most breastfeeding mothers sleep with their knees pulled up and their arms above the baby's head).

It's worth being aware that many parents find it hard to persuade the baby, as it grows into a toddler, to move to its own bed. If another baby comes along making the move essential, this can cause added stress. However, if you're aware of this potential problem you should be able to plan for it, and there's no reason why the move can't be straightforward. Again, some points for and against.

Pros	Cons
You can't get closer to the baby when you're both asleep – and that goes for both parents.	You have to be very careful about avoiding the risks of the baby getting trapped between the bed and the wall.
You can breastfeed the baby lying down.	The risk of SIDS (cot death) is increased if either parent smokes, drinks, takes drugs or sleeps deeply and the baby shares a bed with them.

You can monitor the baby really closely through the night, and respond to its breathing and movement patterns.	All the cons above for having the baby next to your bed also apply here.
Babies who bedshare spend more of the night asleep than those who sleep alone.	

OTHER POINTS TO CONSIDER

- The *number* of pros or cons in the list above is not a particularly good guide to help you make the decision. It's the *nature* of the pros and cons that counts.

- Remember that whichever room the baby is in at night will need to have space for nappy changing and all the absurd amount of gubbins that goes with it, unless you swap rooms to change the baby's nappy. This may wake one or both of you up more than you'd like.

- You won't want to be too far from the bathroom. The water supply can be handy for clearing up the worst nappies – and when you're half asleep is already not a good time for doing this, without having to trek for miles to get water. Do you take the baby with you (remember, it needs serious cleaning)? Will you leave it behind, probably yelling? If so, where do you feel happy about putting it down? If your house is laid out so that some bedrooms are nearer the bathroom than others, or you have an en suite, this may make a difference in deciding where the baby should sleep.

- If the baby is in another room, so you can't sit up in bed to feed it, you'll need a really comfortable chair to sit in while feeding it.

- Remember that you don't have to put your baby down to sleep during the day in the same room it sleeps in at night.

- If the baby is in another room with a monitor, you'll want to be able to hear it crying even if there's a power cut and the monitor cuts out.

- If you're going to have the baby in your room with you, you'll probably want to keep it there until it's at least six months, or there's not a lot of point in going for that option. You'll probably want to move it to its own room by the time it can climb out of a cot, which is generally between about 12 and 24 months (though some escapologists start training younger than this).

The deadline

You don't have to make this decision until the baby is born, and even then you can change your mind. However, if you're thinking of putting the baby in its own room, and you want to decorate it first (the room, *obviously*), that will bring decision time forward (see *When to decorate the nursery*).

Worst case scenario

The worst case would be if you decide you're not happy with the baby's night time location, in which case you can simply move it. If you're moving the baby further away from you, you may get a couple of nights' griping (depending on how old the baby is) but no worse. So this is not a decision to sweat over.

ASK YOURSELF

- Is your baby in a high risk category for SIDS?

- Are you expecting to breastfeed or bottle feed?

- If you're bottle feeding, who do you expect will be doing the night time feeds?

- How far from your bedroom would the baby's room be?

- How much room is there in your bedroom for a cot or crib?

- How far away from your room or the baby's is the bathroom?

- Are you the neurotic type who won't be able to sleep unless the baby is right beside you?

- Does either of you regularly smoke, drink, take drugs or sleep exceptionally deeply? These all increase the risk of SIDS if the baby shares a bed with you.

- Does either of you regularly need a totally undisturbed night's sleep? Obviously you'd both prefer it, but how essential is it?

- Are you anticipating a caesarean? If so, would you prefer to start off with the baby in your room to minimise the need to go wandering about the house while you're still recovering from the operation?

10

When to start buying stuff

It's so tempting to rush out and stock up on cute baby clothes the moment you find out you're pregnant. And what about cribs and car seats and adorable fluffy teddy bears? Actually though, many people find themselves torn over when to start buying. They daren't tempt fate by buying too soon, but they worry that if they leave it too late they'll run out of time.

The options

Obviously the options between buying the day you do the positive pregnancy test, and the day the baby is due, are all but limitless. However most people waver between starting to buy things:

- in the first half of the pregnancy
- in the middle of the pregnancy
- towards the end of the pregnancy

FIRST HALF OF THE PREGNANCY

Some parents get very excited early on and start buying what they need as soon as possible.

Pros	Cons
It makes the pregnancy feel a lot more real.	There's a huge amount of choice out there, and if you launch into buying sooner than you need, you may waste money on things you never use.
If you're the organised type you'll feel a lot less stressed this way.	If you lose the baby it's likely you'll find it more upsetting if you have already started buying things.

MIDDLE OF THE PREGNANCY

The bulk of parents probably start to buy things at around five or six months. By then the risk of miscarriage is very low, and they are still in good time to be ready when the baby arrives.

Pros	Cons
You still have some energy for shopping.	You may have to resist the temptation to buy things for what feels like a very long time.
You can be pretty confident in the pregnancy.	The earlier you buy the more likely you are to make mistakes, so although this is better than buying right at the start, it's still less reliable than leaving it till later.
You've had some time to decide what you actually want to buy.	

TOWARDS THE END

If you really want to play it safe, and you're pretty laid back about being organised in time, you may prefer to leave the shopping as late as possible.

Pros	Cons
You have the maximum time to decide what you actually want to buy.	If you leave it too late, an early baby could arrive before its clothes do.

The risk of miscarriage is as low as possible.	If you're shopping on foot (rather than by, say, mail order) you'll find it more exhausting the later you leave it.
Giving yourself less time to spend probably means you'll spend less money overall.	

OTHER POINTS TO CONSIDER

- Reports vary, but the cost of a baby up to its first birthday is generally estimated at between £3-5,000. I'd say that most of the money that is wasted (which isn't all of it of course) is spent during the pregnancy. You're probably both still earning at this stage and can afford to spend more.

- There's a frightening array of choice out there, and most of it you can manage perfectly well without, though you may still prefer to have it. There are pieces of equipment that morph into other things (car seats into prams for example) and you'd do well to research the options thoroughly before you make any decisions. In particular, try asking everyone you know with small babies what option they would go for.

- Also find out why your friends would recommend the choices they do. Not everyone has the same requirements. For example, some parents would cite a Moses basket as the single most useful piece of equipment they had while others, with a different house layout/lifestyle/set of priorities, will tell you they bought one and then never used it. These conversations will help you decide what is really worth having *for you*.

- If you want your child's equipment, or the colour of their clothes, to reflect their sex, you can't buy until you know whether you're having a boy or a girl. This may prompt you to ask at your scan (if your hospital will tell you) or to delay buying as much as possible until after the birth.

- Remember that you can shop online or by mail order as well as in town centres. A quick internet search, or asking friends who have babies, will reveal a wide selection of excellent mail order companies. Some things are better bought this way than others, mind you. The key things when buying a pushchair or buggy are testing the handlebar height for comfort, and practising folding and opening it to see how easy you find it. You can't do that online.

- Bear in mind that baby clothes that say 'newborn' or 'up to 1 month' are too small for many big babies from the start. Even if your baby is an average size these clothes will be worn only a few times before they're outgrown. To avoid wasting money it can be a good idea to buy clothes that say '0–3 months', unless you know your baby is going to be small. Someone gave me this advice during my first pregnancy and I was extremely grateful for it when the baby turned out, without warning, to be almost 10lbs.

- Most couples find that they're offered lots of things by friends and family, either as gifts or second hand. It's worth finding out what you're going to be given *before* you go out and spend a fortune.

- If you don't want to tempt fate by buying too soon but you find it hard to resist, you might allow yourself to buy just one thing really early on.

- Chapter 12 gives you more information about what is really essential to buy.

The deadline

Quite clearly the object of the exercise is to make sure you have everything you need by the time the baby is born. However bear in mind that there are lots of things you don't need until after the birth. For example if you use a baby carrier you may not need a pushchair for a while. And the baby won't be able to hold so much as a rattle for several weeks.

Worst case scenario

The worst case scenario – apart from not being able to get in through your front door for baby clutter – is obviously that you buy the stuff and then miscarry. Only you know how this would make you feel.

At the other end of the scale the danger is that the baby will arrive before you have everything ready. Bear in mind that not having bought a baby gym yet is not life threatening. Family will rally round and nip out shopping for you, friends will give you cast-offs, and the baby will be fine. The biggest risk is to your stress levels if you're the type that gets stressed by not being prepared. But the risk to the baby is nil.

ASK YOURSELF

- How will you feel if you start buying stuff and then miscarry?

- How will you feel if the baby arrives before you've bought everything?

- What clothes and equipment will you be given by friends and family?

- What do you need now and what can wait until after the baby is born?

- How tight is your budget – now and once you're on leave?

- Have you done your research into the expensive items to be sure you don't buy anything you won't get full value from?

11

When to decorate the nursery

Sooner or later your baby is going to turn into a child that needs its own bedroom. Even if it sleeps with you for the first few months you may still want a room it can play in, and maybe nap in, during the day. And before too long it will be sleeping there at night too.

Whichever room you decide to allocate as the nursery is probably not already decorated in baby pink or blue, with pretty mobiles hanging from the walls and a cot ready in the corner. It's more likely to be full of boxes with a desk covered in bills squeezed into the corner, or maybe it's a spare bedroom doubling with an overflow wardrobe. So something needs to be done to convert it into a charming nursery before the baby arrives.

The options

Most people opt to get the nursery sorted out as soon as possible, though without rushing this means it may take several weeks or even a few months, or they leave it until late in the pregnancy (say around seven months) just in case something goes wrong. So your likely options are:

- do it now
- save it until late pregnancy

DO IT NOW

It's very tempting to get on with organising the nursery as soon as you've decided where it will be.

Pros	Cons
You'll have plenty of time to do it without getting stressed.	If the pregnancy fails, you're likely to find it upsetting having the nursery there.
Any paint fumes will have cleared well before the baby is born.	You may be less sure what equipment you want at this stage.

It's exhausting decorating when you're heavily pregnant (although if you're a couple one of you won't be heavily pregnant, and will therefore end up doing all the work if you leave it till later).

SAVE IT UNTIL LATE PREGNANCY

Logistically, it makes sense to get the nursery organised reasonably early on, before you get too tired, and then leave yourself plenty of time to buy up the odd baby nightlight here or cushion cover there. The argument for leaving it late is that it can be especially traumatic if you lose the baby when you have a nursery all ready and waiting.

Pros	Cons
You minimise the risk of losing the baby and then having a constant reminder of its absence.	You may get stressed if you push the deadline too close.
You're more likely to have worked out what equipment you need.	You may find yourself rushing decisions you didn't want to, for example if you can't find curtains you like.
	Ideally you don't want paint fumes in the house when the baby arrives.
	It's harder work decorating, and shopping for the nursery, if you're heavily pregnant.

OTHER POINTS TO CONSIDER

- If you need to do any building work to create a nursery (converting a garage, partitioning one room into two) it's worth doing this early on even if you don't turn the resulting shell into a nursery until later. Any kind of building work is stressful and especially so when you're pregnant. You'll be wanting to nap without the sound of hammering, and you'll run out of energy to help or oversee. And the deadline of the baby's birth is immovable, so if you leave the building work until later you're likely to find it very stressful if it overruns.

- If you don't want to tempt fate by decorating until later, you can still clear the designated room early in the pregnancy. If anything were to go wrong you wouldn't have any baby clutter around to upset you, and that room could probably do with a tidy out anyway.

- If you choose to decorate the nursery in pink or blue to suit the girl or boy you know you're expecting, bear in mind that if you have another baby and want to put it in the nursery, you may have to redecorate. Likewise motifs such as fairies and space rockets may not turn out to be very unisex.

- Paint fumes aren't pleasant when you're pregnant, and they probably won't be good for the baby. You can get low odour non-toxic paints which are a good idea. If, dutifully following sod's law, they fail to come in the colour you want, it's a good idea to paint the nursery a month or two ahead of the baby's due date.

- I have decorated when heavily pregnant and it's perfectly possible, but actually it's more fun to put your feet up and get someone to make you a cup of tea. There is a nesting instinct in late pregnancy which you can put to good use in the new nursery, but ideally it's better to use it for soft furnishings and the like, and have the heavy work (and anything that involves going up a ladder) out of the way by around six or seven months.

- Remember that even if you have done nothing before the baby arrives, it's not the end of the world. The baby's birth tends to loom as a cut-off point beyond which the world will cease to turn on its axis and anything that hasn't been done already never will be. But actually, you will still be able to buy a nightlight or hang a set of curtains after the baby arrives.

- When you're planning the nursery, don't forget the safety angle: bookcases and so on should be very stable, and fixed to the wall if there's any scope for them to be pulled down. Any electrical sockets and fittings should be out of reach. These things aren't a risk with a newborn baby, obviously, but now is the best time to get them in place.

- Remember that babies are clutter magnets. You need to allow room for about a hundredweight of fluffy toys which they'll assemble in the first few months, a ton of other toys, and a wardrobe that Imelda Marcos would have trouble filling. Over the next couple of years they'll also acquire mobiles, wall hangings, pictures, child's furniture and a library of books. So you need to start with a fairly minimalist look if you're to have any hope of accommodating everything over the next few years.

- Allow space for changing your mind about equipment if you can. For example, you may think you don't need a baby changing space in the nursery as you'll always do it in your bedroom or your living room. But you may find when it comes to it that you do want to change the baby in the nursery. So you'll need room for a mat, a stash of nappies, cotton wool and so on. Or you might plan for the baby to play in the living room and then find you need more room for toys in the nursery than you'd anticipated. Many parents find that their advance plans alter when the baby actually arrives, so try to leave yourself room for manoeuvre.

The deadline

You need the nursery ready by the time the baby moves into it. This may be as soon as it's born, but it may not be until it's six months or a year old, perhaps even more.

Worst case scenario

The worst thing has to be losing the pregnancy after you have the nursery all ready and prepared. At the other end of the decision options, having the baby before the nursery is ready is stressful for some people (though not for all) but isn't life threatening.

ASK YOURSELF

- How much work do you need to do to prepare the nursery? Are you converting part of the house or just slapping a lick of paint round a spare bedroom?

- How would you cope if you prepared the nursery and then miscarried?

- How would your stress levels cope if you didn't have the nursery ready when the baby arrived? What if you hadn't started work on it? What if it was decorated but a few furnishings weren't bought?

- Who is going to do the work? Will you get someone in or will you be doing the work yourselves?

- Do you need a budget?

- Do you want to know what sex the baby is in order to choose a scheme for the nursery?

- Are you sure what equipment you'll need in the nursery?

11

What to buy before the baby is born

You'll be deluged with advice about what you need, from brochures, magazines and shops, and from friends who swear by this or that piece of equipment. Once the baby has arrived it's a bit easier to judge what you need. But buying equipment for a baby when you've never had one before is a bit like packing for a holiday when you don't know where you're going (will I need sun cream? a ski suit? foreign currency? jabs from the doctor?). Sure, you can pack everything, but it will weigh a ton, cost you a fortune and most of it won't be used.

The options

This is a how long is a piece of string question. But the two extreme points that you're likely to fall somewhere between are:

- buy only the essentials until the baby arrives and buy anything else as you need it
- buy everything before the birth so you know it's there when you need it

BUY THE ESSENTIALS ONLY

The budget approach is to buy only what you know you're going to need up until the baby is a week or two old, and save all the rest of the shopping for later.

Pros	Cons
This will save you money in the long run as well as the short run as you'll make fewer mistakes.	You may find you've missed something you wish you had bought in advance.
It means there's less to prepare during pregnancy, which is good if you're feeling tired and uncomfortable.	You'll have to make more shopping trips later – with a baby in tow – to buy equipment.
Your house won't be cluttered with baby stuff.	

BUY EVERYTHING BEFORE THE BIRTH

At the other end of the scale, you can buy everything you could need for the first few months or so of the baby's life, and be fully equipped before the birth.

Pros	Cons
You can't possibly find yourself caught out without something you need when the baby is born.	This inevitably costs you more, and you'll end up wasting money on things you never use.
You won't actually need to leave your house for several months after the birth; at least, not on the baby's account.	You'll be lucky to find anywhere to put the baby down when you get it home as there will be clutter everywhere.
	You may find the shopping very tiring, especially if you leave much of it towards the end of the pregnancy.

WHAT ARE THE ESSENTIALS?

If you're wondering what you absolutely have to have when the baby arrives, the list is shorter than you might think, especially compared to what many baby equipment companies, magazines and friends may have you believe that you need. There's more information in the companion volume to this, *Babies for Beginners*, but here's a quick list of what you really, really need:

● nappies

● cotton wool (or baby wipes)

- something for the baby to sleep in
- baby bedding
- a car seat, if the baby is ever going to travel by car (eg going home from the hospital)
- clothes

And if you're going to be bottle feeding you'll also need:

- bottles with teats and caps
- sterilising equipment
- formula milk
- a kettle (you probably have one of these already)

Not many people would want to manage on this little equipment, but the point is that it's perfectly possible and will do your baby no harm. You can bath it in a bucket or in the sink (mind its head on the taps), and dry it with your own towels.

In addition to this, you will find the following extremely useful, though not essential:

- a changing mat
- some kind of transport for the baby: a sling, buggy or pram
- bibs
- clean-up cloths of some kind
- nursing bras if you're breastfeeding

Of course almost everyone buys more than this, but it's a useful reminder of how little is really essential.

OTHER POINTS TO CONSIDER

- It's well worth setting a budget, even if you're lucky enough not to have to. As well as helping prevent overspending, it encourages you to think hard about what you really need. It's not only money you need to consider – space is often a big issue with baby equipment, and it is preferable to have room in the house for you and the baby, rather than cram it so full of car seats, buggies, baby gyms, clothes and all the rest that you guys have to sleep in the shed.

- Unless you live dozens of miles from the nearest shops, it's really not a hassle going out to buy equipment after the baby is born. In fact it makes a perfectly pleasant trip with a baby. It will probably sleep in the car or buggy on the way there, and baby shops always have decent changing facilities.

- What you think you're going to need, and what you actually need, *never* tally. Some parents get closer than others, but everyone has at least something they bought and never used. And almost invariably it's something they bought before the baby was born. Ask your friends with kids if you don't believe me.

- Remember that most babies around the world, and throughout history, survive happily without most of the equipment you're often told you 'won't manage without'. Be aware of the difference between things you need, and things you merely want because they make your life easier or more comfortable. That doesn't mean you shouldn't buy the latter, but it's less stressful to manage without if you recognise that these things really aren't essential.

- Beware of that dangerous psychological trap of thinking that the world stops when the baby is born. It's easy to convince yourself that you must have everything ready before the baby arrives, as though you were preparing for a long stay in a nuclear bunker. If you're the kind of person who thinks like this (and I can totally get behind that view) try to set yourself more than one deadline. By the birth I need to have x equipment, and by the time the baby is two months I shall buy y. It can be difficult getting out shopping in the first few days, but by the time the baby is a couple of weeks old you'll be climbing the walls to get out, and a trip to a baby shop is about the lowest-stress trip out there is.

- If the two of you disagree strongly about what is needed, you'll have to come to a resolution. If money isn't tight, can you just buy whatever either one of you wants? If it is, set a budget based on what you can afford. Now can you agree a list of essentials that has to come out of that budget? If any money is left over, move on to your list of non-essentials. Or perhaps any non-essentials come out of your own, rather than shared, finances. Or you could compromise on the bigger spender being allowed to choose a fixed number of items off the non-essential list. Or find a neutral referee you both agree on. There are plenty of ways of solving this: the important thing is that you agree on a broad solution rather than keep fighting over the individual items.

- Unless storage space is an issue it's worth accepting almost any gift that's offered by friends and family. The etiquette is that if they don't want it back for a subsequent child you pass it on to someone else when you've finished with it, assuming you haven't run it into the ground. (Though official advice is that you shouldn't hand on mattresses.) So it won't ultimately be wasted, and you may find it's just what you need.

- Ask your friends what single piece of equipment they were most glad they bought and why. They may not be the same as you, but it's a useful exercise for helping you work out what you really want. (My personal response, should you want to know, would be one of those big horseshoe beanbags that wraps right round you. It's great for supporting your bump in bed before the birth, for taking the baby's weight when breastfeeding, and for putting the baby in when it first starts to sit up.)

The deadline

The deadline for each piece of equipment is when it's needed. It's easy to imagine that the birth is the deadline, but actually there are lots of things you won't need until later. For example many babies don't have a cot, or a buggy, for several months.

Worst case scenario

As is so often the case, the worst thing that can happen is that you lose the baby and find yourself coping with the grief while surrounded by baby equipment.

Apart from that, the problem is finding you need something you haven't got. However you *need* very little and, once the baby arrives, you'll anticipate new needs in plenty of time. For example, if you don't buy a buggy because you're using a baby carrier or sling, you won't suddenly think one day, 'Help! This baby's too heavy. Damn! Why haven't I got a buggy when I need one?' What will happen is that you'll start thinking, 'Hmm. I shan't be able to carry the baby like this for many more weeks. I'd better think about getting a buggy.'

If you go the other way, the risk is finding you've spent several hundred pounds on things you never use.

ASK YOURSELF

- What is your budget?

- How much room have you got to store baby equipment?

- How will you feel if you find you've wasted money on things you never use?

- How will you feel if you aren't fully prepared when the baby is born?

- What equipment do you really need in time for the birth?

- What equipment can wait until you have more idea of what you need?

- If you and your partner disagree about what you need to buy, how are you going to resolve the argument?

- Some people take pride in managing on the basics, while others really appreciate having every last luxury. Whereabouts on the scale do you come?

part three

Decisions about the baby

13

Tests – which ones will you have?

Many parents worry long and hard about which tests to have, if any. There are two basic issues: what if the tests are damaging to the baby, and do you want to know in advance if there are problems? Of course plenty of tests don't raise either of these issues, and most parents have no qualms about the standard blood tests (for anaemia etc), ultrasound scans and so on. It's the tests to establish whether your baby has some kind of congenital illness or deformity that you may be unsure whether to have.

There is plenty of other information about exactly what tests are available, but the questions here are broader: do you want to know if there's a problem? And do you want to know enough to take a risk, albeit a small one, to find out?

The only piece of advice I would give here is that it's a good idea to think these things through before you have the first tests (which won't be before 11 weeks), as you might decide the best option is not to start down the testing route at all.

THE FACTS: TESTS

There are several conditions that would affect your baby that can be diagnosed before birth. These include such things as Down's syndrome, cystic fibrosis or sickle cell anaemia. There are two kinds of tests you can have to help you establish the risk to your baby:

- Non-invasive tests such as scans and blood tests, which will tell you the risk but won't be able to give you a definitive yes or no as to whether your baby is affected.
- Invasive tests such as amniocentesis and CVS, which will usually give you a conclusive answer but which carry some risk to the baby – usually a risk of miscarriage.

Amniocentesis

This test involves a needle being inserted into the uterus to take a sample of amniotic fluid. As the fluid contains cells from the baby, genetic testing can be done on these. It carries a miscarriage risk of around 1%. Amniocentesis is usually done at around 15–18 weeks. Below 13 weeks the risk of miscarriage is higher. The results can take up to three weeks for some conditions (it depends what you're testing for), which is a long time if you're worried, and means that if you choose to terminate on the basis of the results it may be a very late termination. However, for Down's syndrome there is a technique to give you a result within a couple of days (see below).

Amniocentesis is recommended by doctors only if earlier, less conclusive tests have shown up a higher than average risk of some kind of chromosomal abnormality. It is not carried out as standard in all pregnancies. The false positive rate is low (around 1 in 1,000).

CVS

Chorionic villus sampling entails taking a small sample from the placenta to test for chromosomal abnormalities. This test is generally done at 10–12 weeks, and results should take only a few days to come through. On average, CVS is associated with a miscarriage rate about 2.4% higher than normal. However where it is carried out by expeienced staff, the risk of miscarriage is roughly the same as for amniocentesis. If CVS is done before 11 weeks there is a higher than normal risk of severe limb deformities. CVS can also determine the sex of the baby.

The false positive rate (ie a result showing a chromosomal abnormality where in fact there isn't one) is about 1 in 100. If there is doubt an amniocentesis may be recommended to confirm the result. The false negative rate (ie showing there isn't a problem when in fact there is) is about 1 in 1,000.

The options

There are three basic routes you can choose:

- don't have any of the diagnostic tests
- have the non-invasive tests but not the invasive ones
- have all the tests the doctors recommend you might need

DON'T HAVE ANY OF THE TESTS

No one is going to force you to have a test you don't want. You may decide to let your GP or midwife know that you don't want any such tests. This option is quite often taken by couples who have decided that they wouldn't terminate under any circumstances, and therefore they won't take the risk of CVS or amniocentesis.

Pros	Cons
You're not taking the risk of an invasive test.	If there is a problem of any kind you may not know about it until the baby is born.
You're likely to worry less if you've had no negative results (having had no results at all).	If a risk factor shows up in, say, an ultrasound scan, you may not be able to either confirm it or put your mind at rest without an invasive test.
	If you would consider terminating in the event of a severe problem, you won't get the option if you don't know about the problem.

HAVE ONLY THE NON-INVASIVE TESTS

You can choose to have blood tests that will give you an indication of risk, but not go on to have the more invasive tests if the risk is high. If the risk turns out to be low this is a great outcome, but of course the whole point is that you don't know until you get the result. If it turns out to be high, you may end up worrying for months, perhaps needlessly.

Bear in mind that you can delay your decision about going for more invasive tests until you have the results. However if the risk level is shown to be high, and you end up deciding against CVS or amniocentesis, you may wish you hadn't had these tests done at all as you'll simply worry. So it's best to think through all the implications from the start.

Pros	Cons
You're not putting the baby at additional risk.	If the results show a high risk you're likely to worry for the rest of the pregnancy.
If the result is good – ie the baby is at low risk – this is the most reassuring option.	

HAVE ALL THE RELEVANT TESTS

No one is going to recommend you have CVS or amniocentesis without good reason. But if earlier tests show a high risk of some chromosomal abnormality you will be recommended to test further.

Pros	Cons
If termination is an option, this is the only way you'll find out conclusively if the baby is at risk.	You could find that the baby is fine and then lose it to miscarriage as a result of the tests. Keep this in proportion; the risk is about 1 in 100. About 280 pregnancies a year in the UK are miscarried due to invasive testing.

You may not want to terminate but feel strongly that you would want advance warning of any problem. These tests should give you that warning.	Although false results are rare, they can happen. It's worth finding out what the false positive and false negative rates are for the particular tests you've had.

OTHER POINTS TO CONSIDER

- The ultrasound scan at around 18–20 weeks is pretty standard and checks for all sorts of things. Many (though by no means all) hospitals will tell you the sex of the baby at this scan if you want to know it, and it's wonderful to see your baby moving on the screen. Be aware, however, that even if you have elected not to have any tests, you will be told if your scan shows up any significant abnormalities or risks. This can thrust you into the whole testing 'do we or don't we?' scenario unexpectedly.

- The risk level at which you'll be recommended for more invasive testing varies according to your doctor, but generally if the result shows a risk of 1 in 250 or greater you'll be recommended for an amniocentesis. Bear in mind that this result still means that there is a 249 in 250 chance that your baby does not have the condition in question. Of course, you may be told that the risk is higher – maybe 1 in 40. You'll need to balance this risk against the risks and stress of further tests, and against your feelings about having a baby with the condition.

- This is big stuff. You and your partner may have very different views about termination, or raising a disabled child. There is no right or wrong, but you need to discuss these issues and reach an agreement in order to make decisions about testing.

- There may be a risk that if the mother has an infection such as toxoplasmosis or HIV, this can be transmitted to the baby by amniocentesis.

- You may have come across the nuchal translucency scan for Down's syndrome. This is usually done between 11–13 weeks if there is a high risk of Down's. It is an ultrasound scanning technique that measures the amount of fluid at the back of the neck. This cannot give a definitive diagnosis, it can only tell you if there is a high risk. A blood test as well as a nuchal translucency scan (known as the combined test) will give you a more accurate indicator of risk. If it is high, you'll be recommended to have an amniocentesis.

- The risk of Down's syndrome (the most common chromosomal abnormality) increases according to the mother's age. Before taking other factors into account, the risk for a 20 year old is 1 in 1,600 while the risk for a 45-year-old mother is 1 in 30.

- Doctors and midwives vary enormously, of course, but broadly speaking the medical profession is geared to establishing diagnoses. So if you simply go with the flow, the system will tend to carry you along in the direction of having blood tests and, if the results show a significant risk, following these with a more invasive test. Some doctors may even carry out diagnostic blood tests alongside other blood tests without checking with you first. So if you don't want to go down the testing route, it's a good idea to make sure your GP and midwife know this.

The deadline

The doctor or midwife will talk you through when the various tests will be offered. Generally speaking the normal times for testing are:

- 10–12 weeks: CVS

- 11–13 weeks: nuchal translucency scan

- 11–20 weeks: blood tests

- 16–18 weeks: amniocentesis

- 18–20 weeks: ultrasound scan (some health authorities also offer ultrasound at around 13 weeks)

Worst case scenario

This depends on what you consider worst, and some scenarios below might not be dreadful to you, but the scenarios to consider are:

- You have a baby with severe problems without any warning through not having done any tests.

- You spend all pregnancy worrying about a high risk but without being able to confirm or refute it as you don't want the invasive tests.

- You have CVS or amniocentesis which shows your baby is healthy, but it then miscarries as a result of the testing.

ASK YOURSELF

- If your baby had a severe disability, would you want to terminate the pregnancy?

- If you wouldn't terminate, how strongly do you want to know in advance if there is a severe disability?

- How much of a worrier are you? If you had the non-invasive tests and they showed a high risk, would that ruin the pregnancy for you unless you had a more conclusive – and invasive – test?

- Do you and your partner have strong disagreements about either termination or having a disabled child?

For more facts and figures, and unbiased information, about tests I recommend another White Ladder book *How Safe Is Your Baby...?* by Annie Vickerstaff.

14

Should you find out if it's a boy or a girl?

For some reason it's always the big question when you're pregnant, and the first thing you want to know when it's born if you didn't find out before: is it a boy or a girl? In some health areas there's no option of finding out in advance, but if you have the choice of being told at your 18–20 week scan, do you go for it?

Of course, a few parents need to know the answer if there's a high risk of a condition that only affects one sex (such as haemophilia, which affects only males). But for the rest of us it's simply a matter of preference.

Often you're really only tempted to find out because you can. You'd have been quite happy not knowing back in the days when it wasn't an option. And you probably don't fret about not knowing for the first four or five months. But once the possibility of knowing is there, it's just so tempting...

The options

I think we're pretty clear about the choice you have here:

- find out the sex
- don't find out the sex

FIND OUT THE SEX

Even if your local hospital won't tell you the sex of your baby, there's still an option to find out at a private scan if you can afford it. Bear in mind that the result you get can just occasionally be wrong.

Pros	Cons
You'll know what clothes to buy and how to decorate the nursery.	For some people this takes away a lot of the excitement of the birth.

You'll be able to choose a name.	If you're one of the rare cases where the sonographer gives the wrong result, the shock at the birth can be hard to deal with.
You may find you bond better with the baby.	If you miscarry you may find it harder if you've already named your baby and formed a closer bond.
If anyone in the family has strong views on whether they want a boy or a girl (such as an older sibling, a grandparent or, indeed, you) it gives adjustment time.	

DON'T FIND OUT THE SEX

For many parents the traditional approach is still popular. They like to save the discovery of their baby's sex until the birth.

Pros	Cons
There's no risk of getting the wrong result if you don't get a result at all.	You can't plan and buy ahead unless you go for unisex clothes and decorating schemes.
It makes the birth even more exciting.	You have to come up with two names, unless you wait until after the birth to choose a name.
	If you have a strong view on what sex you want your baby to be, you might be very disappointed at the birth.

OTHER POINTS TO CONSIDER

- You and your partner may have very different views about whether to find out the sex before the birth. If this is the case, discuss it and come to an agreement before the 18–20 week scan, or you may not get another chance.

- If you find out the sex of the baby but don't want anyone else to know, best not to let them discover that you know. Otherwise they'll nag you constantly to tell them.

The deadline

Unless you pay to go private, the 18–20 week scan may be your only chance to find out the sex.

Worst case scenario

The two worst scenarios, depending on your personal view, are:

- You find out the sex, form a closer bond with the baby, and then miscarry.

- You feel strongly that you want a boy, or a girl, and don't find out in advance. Then you give birth to the one you wouldn't have chosen.

ASK YOURSELF

- How much do you care whether you have a boy or a girl?

- Is there anyone else closely involved who feels strongly?

- Are there any practical reasons why you need to know in advance? For example, do you want the nursery to be a different colour according to the baby's sex?

- Do you and your partner agree about whether to find out in advance?

- If you were to lose the baby, do you think knowing the sex would make it harder to cope with?

- If you do decide to find out, do you want everyone else to know too?

- If you find out in advance, how would you cope if it turned out that you'd been given the wrong result?

15

Choosing a name

There aren't general options here – just as many choices as your imagination can consider. So this section can't really follow the format of the rest of the book. However, this is often one of the trickiest, and most enjoyable, decisions of your whole pregnancy, and it's one that it's worth giving yourself guidelines for.

Here are some points to consider when you're choosing names.

- Make sure the name you choose will suit an adult as well as a small child.

- Think about how the name works with your surname. Often a long first name goes well with a short surname, and vice versa.

- If your surname begins with a vowel it's usually best to avoid a first name that ends in a vowel sound, as the two tend to run together (eg Mia Anderson).

- Consider any shortened versions of the name. Even if you don't plan to use them, your child's friends will. So make sure you like any shorter versions as well as the full name.

- Think about nicknames as well as shortened versions. Does the name you're considering have any other connotations that might give rise to unpleasant nicknames? If your daughter Nell puts on a lot of weight, she's almost bound to be called Nellie the elephant.

- Think about the initials you're giving your child. If they can be used to tease them at school, unfortunately you can just about guarantee they will be. So think twice before naming your son Peter Owen Ogilvy, or your daughter Dora Olivia Gunning.

- If you have other children you might want to make sure that the names go reasonably well together. It can sound odd to call your children Jane, John and Methusulah.

- Some names, especially those based on celebrities or film characters, can go out of fashion very quickly and date readily. Almost everyone called Shirley was born during the brief period when Shirley Temple was a huge child star, and the name dates them within a few years. If you choose to do this, make sure you like the name for itself and not simply for what or who it represents.

- Many people like to use names that have a family connection. If you can't stand your immediate parents' or grandparents' names, you can always look back further in the family tree and you may find a name you really like.

- Think twice before you give your child a name that is particularly long or difficult to spell. They may curse you all their life every time they have to fill out a form or spell out their name.

QUIRKY NAMES

Many people have strong views on whether or not you should give your child an unusual name. Broadly speaking I've found that people with very normal names are more likely to think it's dreadful to saddle a child with a quirky name, while people who have more unusual names usually think it's a good thing. It's becoming more fashionable to pick unusual names, so your child won't stand out as much, but here are some pros and cons to consider for giving your child a name that gets them noticed.

Pros	Cons
Some research shows that people with more memorable and distinctive names are more successful.	Other research indicates that people with unusual names are less successful.
They will stand out from the crowd.	Their name may be mispronounced or misspelled frequently.
They won't share a name with other people in their class or workplace.	If the name has the wrong connotations or sound it may give rise to teasing at school.
They won't get confused with other people of the same name.	

A couple more points worth considering here:

- Boys are more often teased about unusual names than girls.

- You can always use a more unusual name as a middle name instead of a first name. Your child doesn't have to use this name if they decide they don't like it later.

- Some names are so unusual they're unique – you might have made it up yourself. Other names are very simple and traditional but you very rarely hear them these days. There's no reason why a boy should be teased for being called Jed, for example, or a girl for being called Mab. But they'll almost certainly be the only one in the class. If you want something quirky but are concerned about teasing you could always choose a name from this category. You can even make up a longer version to go on the birth certificate but always call the child by the shorter version. So, for example, Jedron can be universally known as Jed.

Perhaps the best judges of whether it's a good idea or not to give your baby an unusual name are adults who have grown up with quirky names themselves. Bounty, the baby information company, conducted a study of adults with unusual names and found that most, though not all, were happy about it. Respondents gave more than one answer so these percentages add up to more than 100.

- 25% said their name was the main reason they got bullied in the playground.

- 20% chose a nickname to avoid using their real name.

- 11% saw it as a lifelong embarrassment.

On the other hand:

- 62% thought it made them stand out from the crowd.

- 17% thought it would help them go far.

- 58% said they loved their name.

- 67% said they would choose an unusual name for their child.

NAMING TWINS, TRIPLETS OR MORE

If you're expecting twins (or more), you may want to choose names that don't relate to each other particularly, as you would for siblings who are not the same age. However you may prefer to choose names that are in some way connected. If so, here are a few ideas:

- names that start with the same letter, such as Tom and Tabitha

- names that sound alike or are spelled similarly, such as Jack and Zac

- names that follow the same theme such as Iona and Lewis (both Scottish islands), or Lily and Iris

- names which are anagrams of each other, such as Carol and Lorca

- names with related meanings such as Zoe and Eve (Zoe means 'life' in Greek, as does Eve in Hebrew)

WHAT IF YOU CAN'T AGREE?

Sometimes it can be really difficult to find a name that both of you agree on. Obviously you need to find a compromise – here are some ideas:

- If one of you is set on a name the other hates, use it as a middle name.

- If you don't like your partner's choice, can you find a variation on it that you're both happy with? For example if you hate Matilda would you be happy with Tilly – either as the official name or just as the one you always use?

- Or you might both be happy with a different or foreign version of the name – perhaps you don't like Mary but would settle for Marie.

- You could give the child a formal name on their birth certificate but then always use a different name. I've known people put down the name their partner wanted on the birth certificate but then resolutely call the child by a completely different name. It's not a good idea to fall out over this, of course, but for many people it works very well. When the child is older they can make their own decision as to which name they use.

part four

Decisions about the birth

16

Where to have the baby

(home vs hospital)

If you consider having a home birth you'll find the most frequent response you get when you tell people is, 'How brave!' Are you really being brave? And do you want to be? Or do you just want to be in your own house with your own things around you? For some people this is the perfect labour, but others are much happier in a hospital where they feel there is immediate help if anything goes wrong.

THE FACTS: HOME BIRTH VS HOSPITAL

Actually, there's nothing brave at all about choosing a home birth, although currently only around 1 in 50 babies are born at home. Research has shown that home births are at least as safe as hospital births; some studies have indicated that they are safer. (Safety is generally measured in terms of mortality rates for both mother and baby.) This however depends on certain factors if you have a home birth:

- The home birth is planned (which in your case it will be if you're reading this) as the statistics change if you include unplanned home births such as emergency premature labour, or teenagers giving birth without telling anyone.

- You have a qualified midwife in attendance.

- You have access to emergency treatment if you need it (such as a transfer to hospital).

Home births have a much lower rate of intervention (forceps, caesarean and so on) than hospital births. It's worth noting that epidural is not permitted at a home delivery, and pethidine is not always available either.

In one major study, back in 1994, it was found that of those who planned a home birth and began labour at home, 40% of first time mothers transferred to hospital, and 10% of previous birth mothers. Well over a third of these were due to slow or no progress, a quarter due to premature rupture of the membranes, and 15% due to foetal distress.

For more information, research findings and statistics take a look at *How Safe Is Your Baby...?* by Annie Vickerstaff, also published by White Ladder.

The options

The options here are pretty obvious:

- home birth
- hospital birth

HOME BIRTH

Many GPs and midwives will support the decision to have a home birth, but some can be reluctant. You may need to write to the manager of your local community midwifery services if you encounter problems. Or you could use an independent midwife if you can afford it, who will generally charge between £1,500 and £4,000.

Pros	Cons
You have all the comforts of your own home around you, from your favourite pillow to meals when you want them.	If anything goes wrong you may need to transfer to hospital during labour.
You don't have to go through the process of moving from the hospital back home after the birth.	The strongest forms of pain relief aren't available at a home birth.

If you have older children you don't have to leave them.	If you have a busy household you might not want the disturbance of phones ringing and visitors calling to see how it's going.
You can create the atmosphere you want – low lighting, music etc.	One of you is going to have to stay on top of meals, washing up etc for the duration.
You may feel more in control in your own home.	
You are likely (though not guaranteed) to be attended by a midwife you know.	

HOSPITAL BIRTH

The vast majority of births are still in hospital, especially first time births. Even if you opt for a home birth initially, you can change your mind right up to the last minute and go to hospital. Chapter 17 deals with choosing which hospital to use.

Pros	Cons
You have instant access to emergency medical care if things go badly wrong.	You are effectively giving birth in a strange place, and will then probably go back to a ward full of people you don't know whose babies may choose to yell just when yours has finally gone to sleep.
You have access to any form of pain relief including epidural.	You may feel less assertive about having the birth you want when you're not on home territory.

You have more peace and quiet than you might do at home, and visitors only during visiting hours.	You have to get yourself out of the hospital after a couple of days or so and get yourself home.
You can both pretty much get a break from household chores for a few days.	If you have older children you have to leave them while you have the baby, and then return with the new baby in tow.
The midwives may help you with the first nappy change, bath etc, and may even take the baby for a couple of hours if you're getting no sleep.	You have no control over meal times, heating, bedding and so on.
It can be easier to rest and recuperate in hospital without the temptation to get up and look after the house or other children.	Some people just hate hospitals. If you're one of them, this will count against a hospital birth.
	There can be a risk of infection in hospital (MRSA being the most notorious example).

OTHER POINTS TO CONSIDER

- If you are considered high risk for some reason, this doesn't necessarily rule out a home birth so long as you have good access to emergency care. Some studies have shown that a home birth is still safer for all but 'very high risk' mothers, at least when measured in terms of perinatal infant mortality.

- If you set your heart on a home birth and then have to transfer, it can be very disappointing. Much better to check out your local hospital anyway, and know what to expect if you have to go there. That way you'll find it much easier to cope with if you do have to take the hospital option.

- There is a care option you may be able to choose known as Domino, which is short for 'domiciliary, in and out'. Your midwife will look after you at home for the start of labour, then accompany you to the hospital, and then come home with you within a few hours of the birth.

- If you want a water birth, check whether you have access to a hospital with a birthing pool. If not, you'll need to go for a home birth or abandon the birthing pool. If the hospital does have a birthing pool it's a good option for a water birth as you really don't want to have to clean the home pool out afterwards. However, if someone else is using it when you happen to go into labour you won't be able to (obviously – a double labour with a complete stranger and their partner would be a little self-conscious I imagine).

- If you have a hospital birth, you can't get your baby home by car unless you have a baby car seat so you need this before the birth (unless, like me, your local hospital happens to be opposite Mothercare).

- All the evidence indicates that once you have some kind of medical intervention, you're more likely to need more. So for example, an epidural may slow down the labour, which can lead to the need for an assisted delivery (forceps, ventouse etc) or even caesarean. The incidence of post-partum haemorrhage is higher in hospital following such interventions as induction and assisted delivery.

- If you have a home birth, you'll need to be able to make the room warm enough for the baby, and you'll need a phone or mobile signal in case an ambulance needs to be called.

The deadline

If you want a hospital birth you're fine up until the last minute (though see chapter 17 if you don't want to go to your local hospital). If you want a home birth it's best to arrange this by 37 weeks. If you think you may have a fight on your hands getting your GP to co-operate it would be better to start arranging it earlier so you have time to approach your community midwifery services manager.

Worst case scenario

Probably the worst thing that can happen is that you start labouring at home and then find you need to transfer to hospital. This isn't likely to cause medical complications but it's a pain.

ASK YOURSELF

- How important is privacy to you?

- Do you feel intimidated or reassured by being surrounded by medical equipment and professionals?

- Does the idea of medical intervention (forceps, caesarean and so on) in the event of a problem labour make you feel better or worse?

- What level of pain relief are you hoping to use (more on this in chapter 18)?

- Do you have older children? Do you feel strongly about whether they'd want you around during the birth?

- How assertive are you? Do you feel confident you can get your view across during labour regardless of whose territory you're on?

- Is your house likely to be empty or full of visitors when the baby is born? Does your answer to this question make you want to be there or want to escape?

- How do you feel about hospitals?

17

Choosing a hospital

If you can't stand your consultant, or hate the local hospital, you have the option of giving birth in a different hospital. So how do you choose?

The options

If you live in a rural area you may not get much choice about which hospital to use. However, in some areas such as big cities there may be several hospitals to choose between. You have the right to be treated at the hospital of your choice. In addition to the choice of hospital, you may also have the option of having your baby in a birth centre. So I'll look at these options against each other:

- birth centre
- hospital

BIRTH CENTRE

A birth centre is sort of half way between home and hospital: it's a small maternity unit staffed by midwives. It is relaxed and homely, and may well have a birthing pool, massages, complementary therapies and so on. Birth centres cannot offer the interventions you can get at a hospital, so usually no epidurals, assisted deliveries or caesareans. If the labour runs into problems you'll be transferred to hospital. The number of birth centres around the UK is growing, so there's a good chance this could be an option for you. NHS birth centres are free, and there are also private birth centres which will cost you around £ £4,000–£5,000.

Pros	Cons
It is very relaxing and comfortable.	Most birth centres will only allow you to book in if you are classed as low risk.

Fewer interventions mean you are less likely to need further interventions such as assisted delivery, episiotomy, induction or caesarean.	If you encounter problems you will have to transfer to hospital.
You will generally have the same midwife with you throughout your labour.	
Post-natal care and breastfeeding support are excellent.	
You will generally be encouraged to stay in for longer after the birth until you're ready to go home.	

HOSPITAL

The last section looked at the pros and cons of hospital births in general; this is a list of the pros and cons of choosing a hospital birth instead of a birth centre.

Pros	Cons
If you are medium risk or above you will probably not have the option of a birth centre.	Your midwife will change whenever the shifts change. Fine if you have a very short labour, but for a long labour you may get several changes of midwife.

If the birth becomes difficult and you need intervention, you're in the right place.	While some hospitals offer good post-natal and breastfeeding support, this is patchy compared with birth centres, which pride themselves on excellent help after the birth.
	A hospital won't be as homely and relaxing as a birth centre.

CHOOSING A HOSPITAL

If you decide that you want a hospital birth, and you have a choice of hospitals nearby, how will you pick the one you want to use? You certainly need to visit any hospitals you are considering using, and talk to the staff to get a feel for how they do things. Here are a few more things to think about:

- How close the hospital (or birth centre) is to your home.

- Which staff strike you as being the most friendly and helpful.

- What extras they offer, such as a birthing pool, private rooms, or anything else you think you might want.

- What their attitude is to any potential complications you think might apply. For example, if you're expecting twins you might feel strongly that you want a natural birth. Some hospitals deliver twins by caesarean as standard, while others will have a more flexible policy than others over this.

- How amenable they are to any forms of complementary treatment you might want, such as acupuncture or aromatherapy.

- How long you can stay after the birth.

- Ask for the hospital's statistics on anything that matters to you: caesarean births, average length of stay after the birth, induction rate and so on.

OTHER POINTS TO CONSIDER

- Some hospitals with birthing pools will not allow you to give birth in the water. If this is important to you, check this out with each hospital or birth centre you're considering.

- The length of time you stay in hospital after the birth depends largely on the kind of labour and birth you have. Around one in six women leave hospital on the same day as the birth, and over a third leave the next day. If you have a caesarean you'll probably be in hospital for at least three days and maybe longer.

- Remember to ask any friends in the area what choices they made and how they felt the hospital or birth centre performed.

- In certain areas, where one hospital offers better antenatal care and another is nearer or has better facilities for delivery, you can book into one hospital and then switch to the other towards the end of the pregnancy. Obviously this isn't hugely popular with the midwives and other staff as it increases their paperwork, but it's your right to choose where you give birth.

The deadline

There's no legal time limit to make your decision, though obviously if you make a last minute decision all the bureaucratic machinery may not be in place (such as maternity records and so on). In any case you'll probably want to make this decision at least a couple of months before your due date.

Worst case scenario

The worst that can happen is that you end up in a hospital that you're not happy with. However with good planning that shouldn't happen and, even if it does, it shouldn't detrimentally affect your baby's health or your own.

ASK YOURSELF

- What are the options in your area?

- How likely are you to need medical intervention? For example, are you classed as high risk, or do you plan to ask for an epidural?

- Do you qualify for a birth centre (ie are you classed as low risk)?

- How long do you think you want to stay in after the birth (see chapter 23)?

- Do you want a lot of support with breastfeeding?

- How important to you is the atmosphere when you're in labour?

18

What kind of pain relief to have

Obviously you don't always get a choice about every detail of your labour. But it does help to go into the labour with some idea of how you'd like to go through it in an ideal world. Some people know they want to use a TENS machine, for example, or plan to ask for every painkiller known to womankind. Although the reality may not match exactly what you'd hoped for, this guide should help you revise your decision if you need to when the time comes.

THE FACTS

Just to help you make your decision about what pain relief to plan for, here are a few statistics from the NHS.

- 1 in 5 deliveries is induced.

- 1 in 3 women have an epidural, or a general or spinal anaesthetic.

- 11% of deliveries involve instrumental delivery such as forceps or ventouse.

The options

Some of these options are mutually exclusive; I've indicated where choosing one option effectively rules out another (for example, you can't have an epidural with a water birth). The options you'll find below are:

- no pain relief
- massage
- complementary therapies
- gas and air
- water birth
- epidural
- tens
- pethidine

NO PAIN RELIEF

There's nothing to say you have to have any pain relief at all in labour if you don't want to. Women have gone through labour with little or no pain relief since the dawn of time, and still do in many parts of the world.

Pros	Cons
It's natural.	It might hurt a lot (the only con, but it can be a significant one).
You are more aware of exactly what you're going through.	
There's no danger that you're doing something that might harm the baby.	

MASSAGE

Your birth partner can learn to massage you in the right way to reduce the pain, with slow circular movements to the lower back during contractions. Practise in advance to get the right level of pressure.

Pros	Cons
You can combine it with most other forms of pain relief if you want to.	Some women hate being touched during contractions.
It's non-invasive and can't harm the baby.	It may not give enough pain relief on its own.

COMPLEMENTARY THERAPIES

Many therapies can be used during labour, either alone or along-side other pain relief. These include aromatherapy, reflexology, hypnotherapy, homeopathy, acupuncture and many more.

Pros	Cons
They can be very relaxing and may also significantly reduce the pain.	Some therapies can be hard to accommodate in a hospital setting – it may depend very much on the hospital. At home or in a birth centre it will be easier.
Most of these therapies are non-invasive and can't harm the baby.	You may need a qualified therapist on hand, which isn't always easy to arrange.

GAS AND AIR (ENTONOX)

This is a mixture of oxygen and nitrous oxide which you breathe in through a tube and a mask or mouthpiece. It is available in all hospitals and birth centres, and the midwife will provide it for a home birth.

Pros	Cons
It works quickly.	It makes you a bit light-headed (you may not regard this as a 'con'), but this clears quickly.
You are in control of your own pain relief.	Some people find it makes them feel sick.
	It's painkilling properties are relatively mild.

WATER BIRTH

Many hospitals and birth centres have birthing pools, or you can hire a home birthing pool if you're not planning to go into hospital. Some hospitals allow you actually to deliver the baby underwater while others don't.

Pros	Cons
It's very relaxing and feels very natural.	If you're in a hospital or birth centre and someone else is in the pool first, you may not get the chance to use it.
	At home it can be expensive to hire, and a pain to empty and clean out afterwards.
	You can't use any pain killer stronger than gas and air while in a birthing pool.

EPIDURAL

This is a local anaesthetic that numbs the body from the waist down. It's injected through a small tube into the lower back, and can be topped up if needed as the effects wear off. It has to be administered by an anaesthetist so you have to be in hospital. A mobile epidural delivers a smaller amount of the drug at set intervals; however, the pain relief is less reliable. Either way it will have a significant impact on your labour if you choose to have an epidural.

Pros	Cons
It gives total relief from pain for over 90% of women.	As you're numb, you have to stay in bed once an epidural has been given. You are effectively disabled for your labour. This makes it incompatible with a water birth, among other things.
	Your bladder will also be numbed, so you will need a catheter to pass urine. You'll also be hooked up to various other drips and monitors.
	As you can't feel when you need to push, labour may take longer and you're more likely to need an assisted delivery such as forceps or ventouse. One in ten women who has an epidural will go on to need a caesarean she wouldn't have had using some other form of analgesia.
	The drug can enter the baby's system so its heartbeat will need to be monitored during labour. Around 10% of babies experience a serious abnormal heart rate episode following an epidural.
	Up to 15% of women have a fever following an epidural – the longer the labour, the higher the risk. This can lead to your baby being given tests and preventive antibiotics.

	About 1 in 1,000 women suffer a severe headache following an epidural, usually because the needle hasn't gone into quite the right place.

Spinal anaesthetic is an alternative to epidural. It is a one-off injection into the spine (obviously) which gives pain relief for about two hours. It's most commonly used for assisted deliveries and caesareans where a very strong block is needed.

TENS

A TENS machine, which can easily be hired if your hospital or birth centre can't provide one, has two pairs of stick on electrodes which you attach at the base of your spine. You can then control the strength and frequency of electrical impulses that block out the pain message to the brain. You're advised to use the TENS machine for a few weeks leading up to labour for best effect.

Pros	Cons
It's a non-invasive method of pain control that can be effective, especially for second and subsequent labours.	You obviously can't use a TENS machine underwater so it can't be combined with a water birth.
You control the machine, which puts you firmly in charge of your own pain control.	The pain relief may not be strong enough for you.

PETHIDINE

This is an injection given into the buttock which gives pain relief that lasts for three to four hours. Diamorphine is a more recently introduced alternative to pethidine. It is also an opiate and acts in a similar way, but seems to have fewer side effects.

Pros	Cons
It's stronger than gas and air or the other forms of pain relief above.	It can make you feel drowsy and therefore not fully in control.
It is also a sedative so in a long labour it can help the mother to rest.	It often causes severe nausea. For this reason it's often mixed with an anti-emetic.
	It's not advised close to the time of delivery as it will cross the placenta and enter your baby's system. This can make the baby drowsy and slow its ability to breathe spontaneously.

OTHER POINTS TO CONSIDER

- Do try to prepare yourself for the possibility that you won't get the labour you'd hoped for, especially if you're planning a low intervention labour. Things do go wrong and many women are understandably very disappointed if they'd hoped for a water birth, say, and end up with an epidural. It can be hard to prepare, but at least make sure you know what the alternatives are so that you can still make an educated decision. And visualise yourself having an epidural so it seems less alien if it happens.

- The midwife will talk you through the options as your labour progresses. Most midwives will be very sympathetic to your wishes, but be clear about what you want and understand the options as the occasional midwife may try to pressure you into an option you don't want to take.

- Not all hospitals offer a 24 hour epidural service. If you think you might want an epidural it's a good idea to check this out with your hospital so at least you're forewarned.

- The attitude you start your labour with can make a big difference. Of course that's easy to say and harder to control. But many midwives report that you can generally tell how well a woman's labour will go as soon as she walks into the room. If her attitude is positive – 'I know it's going to hurt but it will be worth it, and I can take it' – the labour is usually a good one. If she starts out saying, 'I'm terrified this is going to be agony; get the epidural ready NOW,' the labour is likely to be tough. Of course some unlucky women start out positive and end up with complications that make labour difficult, but it's a good rule of thumb.

- If you're the type to be easily worried, try not to listen to all those people who will delight in telling you horror stories about their/their friend's/their sister's labour. As soon as they start just be assertive and say, 'I don't want to hear any negative labour stories, thank you.'

The deadline

You can change your mind at any moment in the labour ward, but you will need to organise in advance if you want to hire a home birthing pool or a TENS machine as you'll need to book them at least a few days ahead.

Worst case scenario

The worst that can happen is that it will hurt a lot more than you'd bargained for. However most pain relief can be provided very quickly, so at any point you can shout, 'That's it. I can't take any more!' and someone will do something about it for you.

ASK YOURSELF

- What is your pain threshold like?
- Do you have strong views about natural birth?
- Do you have any clear feelings about what kind of pain relief you want?
- Are there any medical factors that lead you to think the birth will be either easy or problematic?

19
Who will be at the birth?

It's entirely up to you who is at the birth with you, if anyone. Most women choose their partner but some are unable to or don't think their partner would be any use, and prefer a friend, their mother or a doula (see below). Research has shown that women who have a supportive birth companion are less likely to need major medical intervention such as a caesarean, so there's a good reason to have someone with you who you think will help.

The options

The key options you have for a birth partner (as it's often known) are:

- your partner
- your mother, sister or a friend
- a doula

YOUR PARTNER

According to recent surveys, nearly nine out of 10 fathers attend the birth of their child. However sometimes there is no partner by the time of the birth, or they cannot attend for some reason. And some men prefer not to be there, or the mother doesn't want them there.

Pros	Cons
It's their child too, and they may want to see its first moments.	Some men find it hard to view their partner sexually after watching her give birth.
They will have your interests at heart better than anyone if there are decisions to be made.	Some women feel their sex life will be affected by having their partner watch them give birth.
	Just because your partner loves you, it doesn't automatically follow that he'll be any use at the birth. If he's very squeamish, or under-assertive, he may not be the best person to support you.

YOUR MOTHER, SISTER OR A FRIEND

Not all birth partners have to be women, but unless the father is with you it is the norm. It also gives you the advantage of being able to choose someone who has been through it themselves.

Pros	Cons
Your mother has been through labour herself or, if you pick someone else, you can choose someone who has children.	The baby's father may feel he is missing out on the birth of his child.
If you don't want your partner to witness you giving birth, this is a good alternative.	This is not a good moment to start finding that your own family irritate you. If your sister always winds you up, or your mother makes you feel like a small child, don't assume this will change in the labour ward. You don't want to start a family feud.

A DOULA

A doula is a paid helper who is not a medical professional but who has had a baby themselves and will support the mother around the time of the birth. They can be employed full time or part time, and will help after the birth as well for weeks or even months – according to how long you choose to employ them for.

Pros	Cons
Recent research indicates that having a doula at the birth can reduce the likelihood of medical interventions such as assisted delivery and caesarean.	You will get to know your doula before the birth, but she won't be as familiar as your own family.
A doula is experienced as a birth partner so will know how best to support you.	

OTHER POINTS TO CONSIDER

- While the midwives might get a bit shirty if you try to hold a party in the labour room, you should be able to have at least a couple of birth partners if you want. Check with your midwife if you plan to have more than one partner and they should be happy to accommodate you.

- Whoever is going to be with you at the birth should be able to attend antenatal classes with you (if you do them) and undertake to be there for the whole labour.

- A large part of your birth companion's job is to be your advocate during labour – as you may not be in a fit state – so they need to understand your wishes fully and be prepared to state your case firmly if necessary.

- If one of you wants the father to be at the birth and the other doesn't, this is a sensitive issue which needs thoughtful discussion. Although the mother is generally seen to be the one with the casting vote, the father-to-be may have good reasons for wanting to be present or absent. Sometimes having a second birth partner as well can help solve this problem.

- If the father-to-be is squeamish, or concerned about his sexual image of his partner, it may be that this can be alleviated by making sure he stays near his partner's head and makes eye contact with her during the birth. Quite honestly this is probably the most useful thing he can do anyway.

- You can be as firm as you like about having only the person/ people you want at the birth. Don't feel pressured into letting anyone come along who you don't really want there. If you feel pressured or on display (in what is actually an extremely private thing) it can slow down the labour. Some labours can speed up nicely once extra 'helpers' have been ushered out of the room.

The deadline

Some people virtually grab someone off the street in an emergency, but broadly speaking you need to make a decision in time for your birth partner to attend antenatal classes with you, and familiarise themselves with your wishes for the birth.

Worst case scenario

The worst option is probably that you end up with no partner at all, in which case you'll still have the midwife. Alternatively, the worst case scenario is that your sex life is detrimentally affected by your partner being present at the birth, or that you fall out permanently with your mother.

ASK YOURSELF

- How supportive do you think your partner will be during the birth?

- How assertive will he be if difficult decisions need to be made?

- Is his sexual attitude to you likely to change as a result of seeing you give birth? It's hard to be sure, but you may well have a pretty good hunch.

- Can he be sure of being available for the birth?

- If you want someone else at the birth instead of (or as well as) your partner, who can you trust to be reliable about turning up to antenatal classes and to the birth?

- If you're considering asking a member of your family, is there friction in your relationship with them? If so, could this come out during the birth?

- Could you afford a doula? Experienced doulas generally cost a few hundred pounds for antenatal care and attending the birth, and charge around £10–£15 per hour for post-natal help.

20

Caesarean or not?

This chapter is about planned (or elective) caesareans, which are the only kind you get to make an advance decision about. Under certain circumstances you may decide that you'd prefer to book into hospital for a caesarean rather than wait and go through with a vaginal delivery.

THE FACTS

Nearly a quarter of women in the UK have caesarean deliveries. In total 9% of deliveries are by planned caesarean.

There are countless reasons why women choose an elective caesarean, including expected complications, multiple births, psychological reasons (perhaps a previous vaginal birth was particularly traumatic) as well as through preference (what the media like to call 'too posh to push'). In most of these cases a caesarian is not essential, though there may be a strong case for it. Ultimately it's your choice.

You don't have an automatic right to a caesarean without a sound medical reason. However you may find that your midwives and doctor will agree to it.

It used to be recommended that once you'd had a caesarean you couldn't subsequently have a vaginal birth, but this is no longer the case. If you decide you want a caesarean this time, it doesn't mean you can't deliver a subsequent baby vaginally - about 70% of such labours are successful.

The options

As we're not discussing emergency caesareans here – which you wouldn't get much choice about – the options are:

- have a caesarean
- don't have a caesarean

HAVE A CAESAREAN

Most planned caesareans are done with an epidural or spinal anaesthetic so that you are awake throughout and can see your baby immediately. Bear in mind that a caesarean is regarded as a major operation.

Pros	Cons
For certain conditions a caesarean is safer for the baby and/or the mother than a vaginal birth.	There is a risk of infection: up to a 34% risk of wound infection according to some studies. Also a 10% risk of urinary tract infection, and risk of bladder damage, chest infection, and thromboembolism, which can lead to thrombosis (the leading cause of direct maternal death).
You know in advance what date your baby will be born.	You can lose a lot more blood than with a vaginal delivery.
It's pain free (at the time – the recovery may be a different matter).	The baby can need extra oxygen to help with its breathing for a few hours (or occasionally longer).
	You'll need to stay in hospital longer, and the recovery will take longer.
	It can be hard following a caesarean to find a comfortable breastfeeding position, although breastfeeding should be perfectly possible.

	The chance of death as a result of a caesarean is tiny, however it is three times higher (for both mother and baby) than for vaginal delivery. That's before you take into account the reasons for having the caesarean, which may outweigh this.

DON'T HAVE A CAESAREAN

Some consultants and hospital midwives are more in favour of caesareans than others (some have rates as low as 13% while others are as high as 30%). If you feel you're being pressured into a caesarean you don't want by a consultant you consider is being over-cautious, you can always see if another hospital nearby is more sympathetic to your view.

Pros	Cons
The risk for the mother is lower.	It can increase the risk to the baby (and sometimes the mother), though it is very rare for a natural delivery to be more risky for the baby than a caesarean.
The recovery period will almost certainly be much shorter.	
On average, women find it easier to bond initially with the baby after a natural birth than after a caesarean.	

The incidence of post-natal depression is lower in women who deliver naturally.	
You won't need to spend so long in hospital.	
It's important to many women to feel they have had a natural birth.	

OTHER POINTS TO CONSIDER

- If there's a case for a caesarean but you opt not to have one, you'll probably be persuaded to have the baby in hospital in any case. If you do this, you should be able at least to have an emergency caesarean if things don't go as you'd planned.

- Some women feel pressured to have a vaginal birth, or feel in themselves that they want a more natural birth. Although it's hard, if there are strong health implications for you or your baby, try to focus on the fact that whether or not you have a caesarean, the important thing is to end up with a healthy baby. It's a huge decision now, but as your child grows up you will barely give a thought to how you delivered them.

- There are lots of medical reasons why a caesarean might be recommended to you. As a lay person it's very hard to tell whether you're being pushed into it by medical professionals who favour intervention generally, or being well advised by someone who only considers caesareans when there are strong reasons. However, you may really want to know this in order to make your decision. To start with, ask what that particular hospital or obstetrician's caesarean rate is. The average at the moment is around 23%. The further above this figure their rate, the more likely they are to recommend a caesarean that others might consider unnecessary. The further below it, the more likely they will only recommend a caesarean with sound reason. However, if their rate is high, it could still be that in this instance a caesarean is the best option. So go online and check out any statistics you can find for the particular problem or condition you have that is causing them to make this recommendation.

• For low risk women, latest findings show that the neonatal mortality rate (ie the mortality rate in babies up to 28 days old) is twice as high in the case of caesarean birth as in vaginal birth (around 1 in 565 as against 1 in over 1,000). The relevance of these findings is that they give a strong indication that it is the delivery method itself that accounts for the increased rate. In high risk women it's harder to assess whether any infant deaths were due to the caesarean itself, or to the medical problem that prompted it.

• The maternal mortality rate for caesarean section is less than 1 in 2,500 (compared with 1 in 10,000 for vaginal delivery).

The deadline

Technically an elective caesarean is any caesarean that is decided on before you go into labour. Often it is a late decision based on complications (such as breech position) that you couldn't have predicted before. Sometimes the reason is one you've known about for many months (such as a multiple birth).

Worst case scenario

There are worst case scenarios whichever way the decision goes. If you opt not to have a caesarean you could end up with serious medical complications, though almost always an emergency caesarean is as bad as it will get. If you choose a caesarean you might not have needed, there is an increased mortality rate for both mother and baby, but bear in mind that the rate is still tiny.

ASK YOURSELF

- What are the risks to your baby or yourself if you don't have a caesarean section?

- Do you have strong personal views either in favour of or against caesarian delivery?

- If you choose to have a caesarean, how will you manage a newborn baby during the recovery period (up to six weeks)? Will you have help?

- Are you happy to spend extra time in hospital (see chapter 23)?

21

What to put in your birth plan

This chapter has a slightly different format from most of the others as there aren't fixed options here. And although there's no need to make a birth plan if you don't want to, there are no positive benefits to not having one. However, what you put in your birth plan is a crucial pregnancy decision so it's worth passing on some advice to help you.

It's unusual, though by no means unheard of, to get *exactly* the birth you hoped for. While it's important to prepare yourself for the fact that all may not go to plan, it's also important to make sure that you have a plan (for it not to go to). Without a plan, you'll get a standard textbook birth. If you want anything different from the norm you'll need to say so. The best way to do this is in writing in your birth plan. When the time comes you may have other things on your mind.

Your midwife should do her best to follow the wishes set out in your birth plan, although of course she may have to advise you to revise your plans if things go differently during labour. But at least she'll know that she's recommending a deviation from your intentions, and she'll be able to explain and advise accordingly. Of course the vast majority of midwives will do their very best to follow your wishes with or without a birth plan, but you'll almost certainly find the process of writing it helps you to think through what you want anyway. Also it may be especially useful to have it in writing if your hospital has a high incidence of some kind of intervention you really don't want.

THE BIRTH PLAN

You may have only one or two points you feel strongly about and want to include, or you may have a long list. It's entirely up to you. Writing a birth plan helps you to focus on what you actually want from the birth so it's a useful process to go through. A comprehensive birth plan will also give your midwife a very good overview of your general approach so they'll know what your attitude is likely to be to other things you've not put in the birth plan. Here are some ideas of things you might want to consider including.

- **Your birth partner.** You can specify who you want with you, and if there are times when you particularly do or don't want them present. Also specify if you want anyone else there, from close family to an alternative therapist.

- **Pain relief.** You can always change your mind when the time comes. But if you have any specific requests, such as trying gas and air alone first, here's the place to mention it.

- **Activity level.** If you particularly want to stay active throughout labour, or want to be in bed, make a note of it.

- **Atmosphere.** If you want any particular music played, or low lighting, say so in your birth plan. You may not always get a choice, but often you will, especially at home or in a birth centre.

- **Birthing pool.** If there's access to a birthing pool, let the midwife know if you'd like to use it.

- **Monitoring the baby.** Do you want occasional monitoring or do you prefer the reassurance of being permanently strapped to a monitor?

- **Induction.** Do you have strong views about whether or not you'd want the labour speeded up and, if so, how? See chapter 22 for more on induction.

- **Birth position.** If you want to give birth in a particular position, mention it in your birth plan and your midwife will be able to prepare you in time when you reach the second stage (ie the stage of labour where you start to push).

- **Assisted delivery.** You might want to express a preference between forceps and ventouse, should it become necessary.

- **Episiotomy.** Do you want to be cut if the midwife or doctor thinks it necessary? There may come a point where they advise you there's no choice, but where they draw the line will be influenced by your birth plan.

- **Delivering the placenta.** Do you want an injection to speed up the third stage (after the baby is born, when you deliver the placenta), or would you prefer to deliver the placenta naturally?

- **Cutting the cord.** Who do you want to cut the cord, and when? The midwife or the father? Straight away, or after the placenta is delivered?

- **Stitching.** Do you want to be stitched should you tear, or do you prefer to heal naturally if possible?

- **Feeding.** Make sure the midwife knows whether you plan to breast or bottle feed, and any other preferences relating to this.

OTHER POINTS TO CONSIDER

- Apparently over 70% of pregnant women in the UK now make a birth plan, so your midwife will be well used to working with one.

- You're likely to feel more confident and in control if you have a birth plan, and able to concentrate on what you're doing without worrying that other details may be forgotten.

- If you have any special needs you might want to include a mention of equipment you'll need or religious requirements that will apply.

- You might be planning a home birth or a delivery in a birth centre. But should things go awry you could end up in hospital. So it's a good idea to include your 'plan B' preferences in your birth plan as well as your preferences for your chosen birth. For example, you might have preferences in the case of an emergency caesarean, or if your baby has to go to the special care baby unit.

- It's an emotionally charged time, and you can find yourself getting emotional about things that may, on paper, not look important in the grand scheme of things. Everyone will tell you that the only thing that matters is having a healthy baby, and you know that makes sense. Nevertheless, not getting to cut the cord yourself, or being induced when it's not what you'd chosen, can be a big deal. You're not being daft - lots of women find they get emotional about the details. That's where a birth plan can really help.

The deadline

You can keep writing your birth plan up until you go into labour. However it's useful to have it written in time to go through it with your midwife before then, in case you have requested anything that might be a problem.

Worst case scenario

If you don't write a birth plan, you may end up wishing later that your birth had gone differently. It won't affect the essential outcome - a healthy baby - but the details can make a difference.

ASK YOURSELF

- What sort of labour do you want? Do you have an image in your mind of how you'd like it to be?

- Do you have any special needs or religious or dietary requirements?

- Do you have clear views about any of the points outlined above?

22

Do you want to be induced?

If your doctor or midwife believes it to be medically advisable, they may recommend that you have your labour induced. This means you will be given either medicine or manual manipulation to break your waters and/or get contractions started. This usually stems from a concern about the health of either the mother or baby and could be offered to you at any point late in the pregnancy, particularly if you are several days past your due date.

Remember, being induced is not a sign of failure by any means. If your baby arrives completely naturally, is induced or requires a caesarean section to be born, it doesn't matter. As long as the outcome is the safe arrival of your child then you've succeeded.

The main reasons for recommending induction are:

- Going beyond your due date
- Waters breaking but no signs of contractions within 24–48 hours
- The growth of the baby has slowed or stopped
- An infection in the uterus
- A lack of amniotic fluid or a drop in levels
- Bleeding during pregnancy
- High blood pressure or pre-eclampsia
- Gestational diabetes
- Detachment of the placenta from the uterine wall

Medical professionals won't recommend induction without a good reason. However it's not an exact science and some midwives and doctors are inevitably more cautious than others. If you don't mind being induced this isn't a big issue, but if you have a strong reason for not wanting to be induced – for example you want the baby at home which is incompatible with induction – you may not agree. Sometimes the midwives will recommend induction but if you see your consultant they may feel it isn't necessary. So you should always take seriously any advice to be induced, but ask for more information and advice if you feel reluctant. For example, I know one woman who was advised by her midwife to be induced as her baby was small for dates. She insisted on a scan first to confirm this – and it turned out the baby wasn't in fact small when measured properly. However had it been so, it might well have been wise to opt for the induction.

The options

- have an induction if medical staff advise it
- don't have one

HAVE AN INDUCTION

There are certainly circumstances when an induction makes sense. Once you have all the facts you may well feel that you want to go along with the advice to be induced.

Pros	Cons
You may know in advance when you are likely to go into labour. This can help prepare you mentally and physically for the arrival of your child.	You may feel psychologically absent from what's happening to your body.
A perfect induction may carry fewer risks than a natural labour for some pregnancies as both the mother and baby are monitored from start to finish.	You will have to be in hospital for an induction.
If you are overdue the risk of an overly large baby or a deteriorating placenta are reduced with a scheduled induction.	Labour can sometimes be fairly fast and furious after induction.

	Unnecessary procedures can lead to difficulties in some pregnancies, such as the requirement of an emergency c-section. Sometimes leaving things to nature is the best policy.

DON'T HAVE AN INDUCTION

If you decide not to be induced you may be given the option to wait until the last minute, but you might also be told that you don't really have a choice. This will depend partly on the reason for it. For example, if you're overdue with no other complications you may agree well in advance the date when you'll be induced if the baby hasn't arrived. I've known this to be as late as 18 days past due date. And you could in theory refuse to be induced at all. However if the reason is, say, threatened pre-eclampsia, which can potentially lead to fatal eclampsia, there may not be much choice. If your condition makes it medically necessary then you do need to be prepared to accept this decision. Having it as an option in your birthing plan can help you deal with this psychologically.

Pros	Cons
You can start and finish your labour at home or in a non-medical birthing centre if you choose.	If you have made your mind up not to be induced and it becomes medically necessary you may not feel in control of your labour and delivery.

Waiting for a natural start to your labour can be less risky for mothers without overriding medical reasons for induction.	Refusing an induction may lead to risks to you or your baby.
If you want to, you can bring on a natural induction yourself through nipple stimulation or ingesting some herbal teas, although these methods are not encouraged and are not guaranteed to work.	

OTHER POINTS TO CONSIDER

- There are several ways in which inductions take place. Not all of these are guaranteed to work. It's possible that you'll be sent home and asked to return in a day or two for another attempt, or that a different method will be used to ensure that labour starts.

- Medication may be administered to you through an IV or suppository to set off contractions. This is usually a synthetic form of a hormone your body produces naturally.

- If your cervix hasn't thinned or softened yet your doctor or midwife may use a procedure called 'stripping the membranes'. This is basically an attempt to separate the placenta from the wall and it is carried out manually during an internal exam. They may also apply a gel or liquid chemical to your cervix to help it soften or use a small balloon filled with water to help it open up.

- If your waters haven't broken then a plastic needle may be inserted and used to make a small tear in the amniotic sac. This leads to the production of prostaglandin, a natural hormone which speeds up contractions.

- While 'stripping the membranes' can lead to an average reduction in labour time of one hour, it can also move babies into the breech position.

- The procedures involved in inductions don't usually hurt, but they may be uncomfortable.

- Inductions, as with natural labours, often take longer with first pregnancies.

- Inductions can be elective, although this is rare.

The deadline

Induction is not an emergency procedure. If the baby has to be got out fast no matter what, you will be recommended to have a c-section and not an induction, as induction is not such an exact science. So you will always be given time to think about induction. You may be advised to be induced within a day or two, or told that it may become necessary in the next couple of weeks. Whatever the timescale, the midwife or doctor will let you know when you need to make a decision.

Worst case scenario

The worst thing that could happen here is that if you opt not to have an induction your health or your baby's could be compromised. This depends largely on the reason for the induction. If you agree to the induction the labour could be faster – which sounds great, and may be just what you want. However a very fast labour can be particularly exhausting and may carry a greater risk of minor but unpleasant side-effects such as tearing.

ASK YOURSELF

- How much confidence do you have in your midwife or doctor?

- Are you happy to have your baby in hospital?

- Are you comfortable about the chance of a speeded-up labour?

- Do you have objections on moral or religious grounds?

- Are you prepared to take the risks of being induced?

- Are you prepared to take the risks of not being induced?

- Are you in a high-risk category?

- Is this your first pregnancy? If not, have you ever delivered by caesarean section?

23

How long will you stay in hospital?

If you choose a home birth, this won't apply. In any case the hospital isn't going to encourage you to stay there indefinitely, occupying a bed and eating their food. But there is some scope for choice, and the choice between birth centre and hospital will also broaden your options.

The options

Most people fall at one end of the scale or the other, so the choices essentially are:

- get out as fast as you can
- stay for as long as you can

GET OUT AS FAST AS YOU CAN

Technically, you can discharge yourself at any time. Realistically, though, the earliest most new mothers leave hospital is about six hours after the birth, and many leave the next day.

Pros	Cons
You can sleep in your own bed and eat in your own kitchen.	You may get more sleep in hospital, as some midwives will take a wakeful baby off you for a little while so you can sleep.
If you hate hospitals this option is for you.	Food is provided in hospital – at home you're on your own. If you don't have much support that can be tough.
If you have older children at home you get back to them quicker.	If you need help looking after the baby you won't get 24 hour a day midwives once you've checked out.
	It's easy to underestimate the amount of help you're going to need if you're breastfeeding. If you can't get the baby to latch on in the early hours of the morning, you might wish you'd stayed in at least for a night.

STAY FOR AS LONG AS YOU CAN

If you have a caesarean section you may need to stay in hospital for up to a week to recover from the surgery. Where there is no medical necessity to stay, you will often still get the option of staying for up to three or four days.

Pros	Cons
You get looked after.	There's very little privacy.
If there are complications you may feel safer.	It can be noisy, too hot and the food may not be to your taste.
You may get more help learning how to look after the baby.	There's some risk of infection.
(You have the company of other new mothers on the ward.)	(You have the company of other new mothers on the ward.)
You'll get help learning to breastfeed.	

OTHER POINTS TO CONSIDER

- Some hospital midwives are very helpful, showing you how to feed and bath your baby. Others may give you little or no help. Once you get home you don't have constant care, but community midwives are almost universally reported to be helpful with these things.

- You are likely to be encouraged to stay longer in a birth centre than in a hospital, as a broad rule of thumb.

- If you think you'll want to stay for a while, ask at your local hospital and birth centre about how long they'll allow you to stay when you're deciding where to have the baby.

- Your hospital isn't going to let you stay forever. However, if you feel unready to go home or you have no help lined up when you get there, they will take this into consideration.

The deadline

You can decide at the time when you feel ready to go home.

Worst case scenario

It's hard to see how staying in too long could be a problem as you can just leave when you feel ready. The worst that can happen is that you check out too soon and then find coping at home is tougher than you were prepared for. It's not the end of the world, but it can give you a pretty fraught night or two.

ASK YOURSELF

- How do you feel about hospitals generally?
- How important is privacy to you?
- How much help will you have when you come out?
- How confident are you about looking after the baby on your own?

24

Who do you want to visit you?

While you are recuperating in hospital there will be dozens if not hundreds of people wondering how you're getting on. Some of them will want to come and visit you and possibly bring lots of lovely presents for you and the baby, but that doesn't mean you have to receive them. If you're feeling up to talking to people then it's your prerogative to choose the ones you want to see, but if you're not feeling healthy or energetic enough it's also perfectly OK to say no.

The options

As this is a very personal decision, there are three options here:

- receive everyone who wants to come and visit you
- receive only a few select people
- receive people only at certain times
- receive no-one other than your birthing partner(s)

RECEIVE EVERYONE WHO WANTS TO VISIT YOU

The nice thing about having lots of people around you after the birth is that everyone is very willing to help you get stuff done. You may be itching to show off your new baby, and having lots of visitors is ideal for some people.

Pros	Cons
Lots of people around you to capture memories and help out if you need to rest.	Little to no privacy.
Visitors can keep your birthing partner entertained while you sleep.	You may feel obliged to stay awake and entertain your guests.
If you're having trouble coping then there are people around to offer you advice.	The advice people offer may not be very welcome at this stage.

| Presents! | There is a small risk of infection to your newborn with added visitors, although this will happen sooner or later anyway. |
| | You may find yourself very protective of the baby, and may be stressed if lots of people are touching it, or indeed being noisy when you think it's sleep time. |

RECEIVE ONLY A FEW SELECT PEOPLE

If you make your choices clear to your friends, family and most importantly, your birthing partner(s), then deciding whom in advance you'd like to visit you can become more selective. It's up to you who gets in, so if you only want your partner, parents and best friend, people will understand.

Pros	Cons
You can surround yourself with people you know love you and your baby unconditionally.	If you really don't feel like having any visitors at the last minute it can be hard to tell close family and friends to stay away.
You can take breaks when you need to rest.	All the cons of having plenty of guests.
Memories can still be captured and people can still offer help and advice.	

You can restrict the visitors to people who you feel comfortable falling asleep in front of, or breastfeeding, or asking to be quiet.

RECEIVE PEOPLE ONLY AT CERTAIN TIMES

You might ask for afternoon visitors only, or ask people not to visit you for the first 48 hours. Or if you have your baby in hospital, you might decide to have visitors for the first day or so but ask to be left alone for the first few hours or days when you go home.

Pros	Cons
You control when you have time alone with the baby.	You may find when the time comes that you want people around for support or company at times when you'd asked them to stay away.
You avoid any particular times you think might be difficult to have visitors, such as the first few hours, or when you first take the baby home.	Some people may be reluctant to follow your guidelines and you may need to be tough with them.
You still have all the benefits of visitors at the times you want them.	

You'll leave plenty of time in your schedule for undisturbed bonding or sleep (well, at least it's only the baby who'll disturb it).

RECEIVE NO-ONE OTHER THAN YOUR BIRTHING PARTNER(S)

This is probably the most delicate of the three options, particularly if you or your partner has a close-knit family who all want to welcome the new addition. You'll need to let people know at what point you will want to see them – you can't keep them away until the baby has grown up and left home.

Pros	Cons
You can focus solely on your new baby and start to heal in peace.	You might upset your friends and family by asking them not to visit.
As it will stay very private, you can ask questions of the medical staff or midwives without embarrassment.	If you change your mind it might be too late for people to book a flight or drive to see you.
There will be no unwanted advice.	

OTHER POINTS TO CONSIDER

- Whatever you decide can be reversed, even at the last minute.

- If this baby is your first, you may not be able to predict how you'll cope with lots of visitors.

- If you do have visitors in hospital, make sure they abide by the hospital's health and safety policy, particularly if they want to handle the baby directly.

- Visitors should also abide by the hospital's visiting hours if you're in hospital, and leave you plenty of time to rest.

- A usual list of visitors might include your partner, both sets of grandparents, a sibling or two and perhaps a close friend. All others can wait a few days until you're settled in at home.

- Young children might be too much to handle at this stage in your healing, unless they're your own.

- The most important factors in your decision are you and your baby. You can afford to be selfish in the first few days if you want to bond in private or with a few select people.

Deadline

This decision can wait until the moment after the baby is born, unless you feel very strongly that you don't want any visitors at all. If this is the case it's probably worth vocalising it about a month before your due date. This will give people a chance to accept your decision and make plans to see you once you've returned home.

> ## Worst case scenario
>
> The worst thing that can happen here is that you change your mind and either feel overwhelmed by all the activity or lonely because no-one came to see you. Either way you and your baby are completely safe from harm.

ASK YOURSELF

- Are you private or outgoing?
- Could you cope with lots of people at one time?
- If you are being selective, who makes the list?
- What happens if something unexpected happened during delivery?
- Do you feel equipped and comfortable discussing it with visitors?
- If you plan on breastfeeding, how do you feel about doing this in a room full of friends and family?
- Will you feel confident enough to ask people to leave if it all gets too much?

What to take to the hospital

Every woman is different, so what you might choose to pack in your hospital bag may differ in some ways from this list. However, there are some things you will find incredibly useful to have with you, so here's a list of the most commonly packed items, along with the reasons for including them.

It's a good idea to have your hospital bag ready to go by about week 36 so that if your baby comes early you're not panicking about where you put your nursing bras or the nappies.

THINGS FOR YOU

- **Sleepwear.** Whether you choose a nightie or pyjamas, you will want something comfortable to sleep in after the birth if the thought of wearing a hospital gown fills you with dread. Bring at least two sets in case one gets dirty during your stay.

- **Socks or slippers.** Hospital floors can get chilly.

- **Dressing gown.** A non-essential, but nice if you get cold.

- **Breastfeeding stuff.** If you're choosing to breastfeed you will want to pack nursing bras and absorbent pads. You'll also want to wear a top that gives easy access for breastfeeding.

- **Underwear and maternity pads.** Disposable maternity knickers are fab for this less than glamorous time, but if you prefer your own pants bring several pairs and some heavy-duty sanitary towels.

- **Toiletries.** This could include your toothbrush and toothpaste, deodorant, shower essentials if that's an option at your hospital, a hair brush, some make-up, lip balm and hand cream. Labour and delivery can be very drying on lips and skin, so it's nice to have something standing by just in case.

- **Make-up and hair dryer/straighteners** etc if you think you'll want these, especially if you're expecting visitors.

- **Normal clothes.** What will you wear to go home in? You probably won't fit into your pre-pregnancy jeans just yet, so bring something loose and comfortable with lots of stretch. Jogging bottoms are perfect.

THINGS FOR THE BABY

- **Clothing.** Everyone has a different idea of 'baby essentials', but generally a babygro and a warm blanket will suffice at the start. Of course, the time of year you have your baby will affect what you dress it in, as summer and winter outfits will be quite different, and you might also choose a special outfit to celebrate your child's arrival at home.

- **Nappy bag.** This will soon be filled with all manner of stuff, but for now make sure you have clean nappies, cotton wool, disposable bags and any supplies you need if you're choosing to bottle feed. Pre-made cartons of formula milk can be extremely helpful in the first few days.

- **Car seat.** OK, you won't actually pack this, but it is something you'll need once the baby arrives if you plan on driving it home.

OTHER STUFF

- **Birth plan.**

- **Prescription medication.**

- **Snacks and drinks.** You may not be encouraged to eat or drink during the later stages of labour, but you'll need to eat during a long labour. Both you and your birthing partner may want something to eat during the event and you will definitely want something once it's over with. You might also want to pack your favourite teabags.

- **Reading material.** If your labour lasts a long time you might want a good book or magazine.

- **Technology.** This could include a mobile phone, camera, video camera, mp3 player or any number of other things to record the birth, share the news and make the whole thing much more enjoyable. Bear in mind though that anything you do bring carries the risk of being stolen.

- **Money for the phone, or a phone card.** Check out what you need at your local hospital, but don't assume they'll let you use a mobile phone on the ward.

- **Notebook and pen.** You might want to commit the whole thing to memory while it's still fresh, or choose to forget everything completely for a while. Either way, it's always good to have a notebook standing by to make notes on any advice the midwives give you.

A final word

I hope I've helped you get through your first nine months of parenthood (the bit before the baby actually arrives) in as relaxed a way as possible, and that you can make confident decisions about your family based on facts and clear thinking, rather than guesswork or biased advice.

It's worth bearing in mind that none of the options in this book is wrong in itself, and that you're mostly trying to choose between best and second best, not between right and wrong. When you're as emotional (and maybe hormonal) as many of us are during pregnancy, details can seem hugely important. But once you have a happy baby safely delivered, you'll realise that how you got there matters less than you thought at the time.

It's not always easy to keep things in perspective, but it helps to recognise that your pregnancy is probably dominating your life at the moment (quite rightly), and once your baby starts growing up it will start to reduce in importance. Remember how you panicked in the run up to your GCSEs, or worried before your driving test? It all seems much less significant now. In the same way, the decisions you make now matter because you deserve a happy, relaxed pregnancy. But making the 'wrong' decision now isn't likely to haunt you for the rest of your life. So it's not worth spoiling an exciting few months worrying.

You've got the facts and you know what decisions you need to make. Be confident and happy, and I hope your pregnancy goes brilliantly and your new child is a delight to you for the rest of your life.

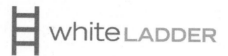

white LADDER

the parenting & family health experts

Get 30% off your next purchase...

We are publishers of a growing **parenting and family health** range of books. We pride ourselves on our friendly and accessible approach whilst providing you with sensible, non-preachy information. This is what makes us **different from other publishers**.

And we are keen to **find out what you think** about our book.

If you love this book **tell us why** and tell your friends. And if you think we could do better, **let us know**. Your thoughts and opinions are important to us and help us produce the best books we possibly can.

As a **thank you** we'll give you 30% off your next purchase. Write to us at **info@whiteladderpress.co.uk** and we'll send you an online voucher by return.

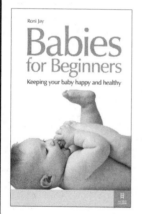
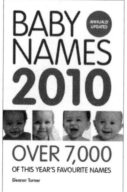
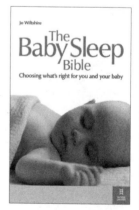

Come and visit us at **www.whiteladderpress.co.uk**